SPANISH FOR ELDERCARE PROFESSIONALS

Language skills for Nurses, Home Health Aides, CNAs and Family Caregivers Working with Spanish-Speaking Elderly Patients

Alessio Ruiz

Educational Use Disclaimer
This guide is intended solely for educational and professional development purposes for eldercare professionals, including geriatricians, nurses, social workers, home health aides, family caregivers, and related practitioners. The Spanish language phrases, terminology, and eldercare scenarios contained herein are provided as learning tools to facilitate communication with Spanish-speaking elderly clients and their families.

Professional Practice Disclaimer
The information contained in this guide does not constitute medical advice, legal counsel, or clinical recommendations. Users must exercise their own professional judgment and adhere to their organization's policies, applicable laws, regulations, and ethical standards when providing care to elderly clients. This material should supplement, not replace, formal training, licensure requirements, supervision, and continuing education in eldercare practice.

Health, Safety, and Language Considerations
Eldercare needs vary significantly across individuals based on health conditions, cognitive status, cultural backgrounds, and personal preferences. Spanish language usage also varies significantly across regions, countries, and cultural contexts. The phrases, terminology, and eldercare scenarios presented may not be universally applicable to all Spanish-speaking elderly populations.
Practitioners and caregivers are strongly encouraged to assess individual needs, verify language preferences and cultural appropriateness with their specific client populations, and seek consultation with qualified interpreters, cultural liaisons, and healthcare professionals when necessary.

Accuracy Disclaimer
While every effort has been made to ensure accuracy of translations, cultural sensitivity, and evidence-based eldercare practices, language is dynamic and evolving, and eldercare knowledge continues to advance.

Users should verify critical communications with qualified interpreters and current standards of care with qualified healthcare professionals, particularly in medical, legal, or crisis situations involving elderly clients. The authors and publishers disclaim any liability for misunderstandings or adverse outcomes resulting from the use of this material.

Ethical and Legal Compliance

Nothing in this guide supersedes professional ethical codes, legal requirements, organizational policies, or regulatory standards governing eldercare practice. Practitioners must comply with all applicable patient rights, informed consent, confidentiality, mandatory reporting, and other professional obligations. Healthcare providers must maintain appropriate licensure and follow scope of practice guidelines. When in doubt, practitioners should seek appropriate supervision, consultation, or specialized services.

Emergency and Crisis Situations

In emergency situations where immediate safety or health is at risk, caregivers should utilize all available resources including emergency medical services, qualified healthcare professionals, and established crisis intervention protocols. This guide is not intended for use in lieu of proper emergency response procedures or immediate medical care.

Continuing Competence and Professional Development

Both Spanish language skills and eldercare knowledge require ongoing practice and refinement. This guide represents a starting point for developing Spanish communication skills in eldercare practice. Practitioners and caregivers are encouraged to pursue additional language training, cultural competency education, specialized eldercare training, and consultation with native speakers and healthcare professionals to enhance their effectiveness in providing quality services to Spanish-speaking elderly clients.

The publishers and authors disclaim all liability for any damages or negative outcomes resulting from the use or misuse of this educational material.

CONTENTS

Title Page

Copyright

Introduction   1

How to use this book   3

Spanish pronunciation essentials   8

Spanish grammar essentials   12

Daily greetings and introductions with elderly patients   19

Asking about comfort and pain levels   21

Explaining daily care routines   24

Building rapport and showing respect   26

Communicating with family members   28

Assisting with bathing and showering   30

Help with dressing and grooming   33

Oral care and dental hygiene   36

Toileting assistance and incontinence care   39

Skin care and preventing bed sores   42

Helping with walking and transfers   45

Using wheelchairs and mobility aids   47

Fall prevention and safety   49

Positioning in bed and turning patients   52

Physical therapy exercises and encouragement   55

Medication reminders and administration 57

Explaining pill schedules 60

Reporting side effects or concerns 62

Managing medication refills 65

Discussing pain management options 68

Meal planning and dietary restrictions 71

Assisting with eating and drinking 74

Managing diabetes and special diets 76

Encouraging hydration 79

Discussing appetite changes 81

Taking vital signs (temperature, blood pressure) 83

Monitoring blood sugar levels 86

Observing and reporting health changes 89

Wound care and dressing changes 92

Recognizing signs of illness or distress 95

Providing comfort during anxiety or confusion 98

Engaging in conversation and activities 101

Dealing with dementia and memory issues 103

Encouraging independence and dignity 106

Managing behavioral challenges 109

Calling for medical help 112

Fall response and injury assessment 114

Choking assistance and first aid 116

Recognizing stroke or heart attack symptoms 118

Contacting family in emergencies 120

Household tasks and light cleaning 123

Laundry and clothing care 126

Transportation to appointments 128

Shopping and errands 130

Managing finances and bills 132

Providing comfort care and pain relief 135

Communicating with hospice teams 138

Supporting grieving family members 141

Maintaining dignity in final stages 144

Cultural and spiritual considerations 147

Recording daily care notes 150

Reporting to nurses and supervisors 152

Communicating with doctors 155

Insurance and healthcare coordination 157

Shift change information sharing 160

INTRODUCTION

The rapidly growing Hispanic elderly population in the United States presents both opportunities and challenges for eldercare professionals. By 2060, the number of Hispanic Americans aged 65 and older is projected to increase from 4.2 million to 18.8 million, representing a dramatic shift in the demographics of those requiring eldercare services. This exponential growth means that healthcare providers, home health aides, nurses, social workers, and family caregivers will increasingly encounter Spanish-speaking elderly clients who may have limited English proficiency or who feel more comfortable communicating in their native language, especially during times of vulnerability, illness, or cognitive decline.

Language barriers in eldercare settings can have serious consequences. When elderly patients cannot effectively express their pain levels, medication concerns, or personal care preferences, their quality of life and health outcomes may suffer significantly.

Cultural nuances in expressing discomfort, family dynamics in decision-making, and respectful communication patterns become even more critical when working with elderly Hispanic clients who may come from traditional backgrounds where formality and respect for authority figures are paramount.

This guide addresses the linguistic needs of eldercare

professionals working with Spanish-speaking elderly clients across all levels of care—from independent living assistance to end-of-life support. Unlike general Spanish phrase books, this resource focuses specifically on the vocabulary, cultural considerations, and communication patterns most relevant to eldercare situations. The content recognizes that elderly clients may use more formal language patterns that differs from contemporary conversational Spanish.

The guide covers eldercare communication thematically, from basic greetings and rapport-building to complex medical discussions and emergency situations.

Special attention is given to sensitive topics such as personal care assistance, pain management, mental health support, and end-of-life care, where language barriers can create additional emotional distress for both clients and caregivers. The guide also acknowledges the important role of family members in Hispanic eldercare, providing phrases for communicating with adult children, spouses, and extended family members who may be involved in care decisions.

Whether you are a healthcare professional seeking to improve patient communication, a home health aide building relationships with clients, or a family caregiver caring for a Spanish-speaking relative, this guide will help you provide more compassionate, effective, and culturally appropriate care. The goal is not to replace professional interpretation services in critical situations, but to enhance daily interactions and build the trust essential for quality eldercare.

HOW TO USE
THIS BOOK

This book is designed for practical, real-world application in eldercare settings, whether you are a complete beginner in Spanish or someone seeking to expand your existing vocabulary for professional use. The book is organized around key areas of eldercare, each containing the essential vocabulary, grammar patterns, practice dialogues, and scenarios you will encounter in your daily work with Spanish-speaking elderly clients.

Structure Of Each Chapter

Every topic follows a consistent four-part format designed to build your confidence and competence progressively. First, the Key Vocabulary section presents the most essential words and phrases for that particular eldercare situation, complete with phonetic pronunciation guides to help you sound confident and clear.

The Grammatical Examples section demonstrates variations in how to properly construct sentences using formal address patterns appropriate for elderly clients. All examples use the respectful "usted" form rather than informal "tú," reflecting the cultural importance of showing respect to elders.

Practice Dialogues provide realistic short conversations between caregivers and elderly clients, showing how vocabulary and grammar work together in natural exchanges. These dialogues model appropriate tone, cultural sensitivity, and the give-and-take of actual eldercare interactions. Practice reading both parts aloud to develop fluency and confidence.

Finally, Practice Scenarios present short stories that demonstrate how language skills apply in real eldercare contexts. These stories help you understand not just what to say, but when and how to say it, including non-verbal communication cues and cultural considerations.

Learning Strategies

If you're new to Spanish, first review the initial pronunciation and grammar sections at the start of the book. Then move on to chapters most relevant to your current role. If you're a home health aide, begin with Basic Communication and Personal Care. If you're a nurse, prioritize Health Monitoring and Medication Management. However, don't skip Basic Communication entirely—establishing rapport is essential for all eldercare relationships.

Use the pronunciation guides consistently that appear in the vocabulary lists at the start of each topic. Spanish pronunciation is more regular than English, so mastering the basic sound patterns will help you with vocabulary throughout the book. Practice the example phrases aloud daily, focusing on clear enunciation and appropriate tone for elderly clients. There's a pronunciation overview at the start of the book if you're new to Spanish along with some grammar tips.

Practical Application

Begin using simple greetings and courtesy phrases immediately, even if your pronunciation isn't perfect. Most elderly clients appreciate the effort and will be patient with your learning process. Gradually incorporate more complex vocabulary as your confidence grows.

Always have backup communication strategies available. Keep a small notebook with key phrases, use translation apps when appropriate, and know when to request professional interpretation services. Remember that this guide supplements, not replaces, proper interpretation in critical medical or legal situations as required by law or policy.

Focus on active listening and non-verbal communication, which are equally important as speaking. Many elderly clients will use gestures, facial expressions, and context clues to help bridge language gaps. Be patient, speak slowly and clearly, and confirm understanding frequently.

Building Cultural Competence

This guide emphasizes cultural appropriateness alongside language skills. Hispanic eldercare often can involve extended family participation in care decisions, sometimes strong religious or spiritual elements and typically specific expectations about respect and formality.

SPANISH PRONUNCIATION ESSENTIALS

Spanish pronunciation is remarkably consistent and predictable compared to English, making it an excellent language for healthcare professionals to learn basic communication skills. Once you master the fundamental sound patterns, you'll be able to pronounce most Spanish words correctly, even ones you've never encountered before. This consistency is particularly valuable in eldercare settings where clear, confident communication builds trust and reduces anxiety for elderly clients.

Vowel Sounds

Spanish has only five vowel sounds, and they never change regardless of their position in a word. This consistency is crucial for eldercare communication, where precise pronunciation can mean the difference between comfort and confusion for elderly clients.

A sounds like "ah" in "father" - always open and clear: "gracias" (GRAH-syahs), "cama" (KAH-mah) E sounds like "eh" in "bet" - never like English "ee": "cliente" (klee-EHN-teh), "pecho" (PEH-choh)

I sounds like "ee" in "beet" - always crisp and short: "medicina" (meh-dee-SEE-nah), "día" (DEE-ah) O sounds like "oh" in "go" - always rounded: "dolor" (doh-LOHR), "socorro" (soh-KOH-rroh) U sounds like "oo" in "boot" - always rounded: "azúcar" (ah-SOO-kahr), "puntos" (POON-tohs)

Key Consonant Patterns

Several Spanish consonants differ significantly from English and are essential for eldercare vocabulary. The rolled R (rr) appears in critical words like "socorro" (help) and "barrera" (barrier). Practice by saying "better, better, better" rapidly, then isolating that middle flap sound. Single R is a light tap, like the middle sound in "better."

C before E or I sounds like "s": "medicina" (meh-dee-SEE-nah), "cinco" (SEEN-koh). C elsewhere sounds like "k": "cama" (KAH-mah), "cuidado" (kwee-DAH-doh). This distinction is vital for medical terms.

G before E or I sounds like English "h": "gente" (HEH-nteh), "giro" (HEE-roh). G elsewhere is hard like "go": "garganta" (gahr-GAHN-tah), "grande" (GRAHN-deh).

J always sounds like English "h": "jabón" (hah-BOHN), "mejor" (meh-HOHR). LL sounds like English "y": "pastillas" (pahs-TEE-yahs), "silla" (SEE-yah). Ñ sounds like "ny" in "canyon": "señora" (seh-NYOH-rah), "año" (AH-nyoh).

Stress And Accent Patterns

Spanish stress patterns follow predictable rules that are essential for eldercare communication. Words ending in vowels, N, or S are stressed on the second-to-last syllable: "enfermera" (en-fehr-MEH-rah), "pastillas" (pahs-TEE-yahs), "medicinas" (meh-dee-SEE-nahs). Words ending in consonants other than N or S are stressed on the last syllable: "dolor" (doh-LOHR), "hospital" (ohs-pee-TAHL), "mejor" (meh-HOHR).

Written accent marks always indicate where to stress the word, overriding normal rules: "médico" (MEH-dee-koh), "sartén" (sahr-TEHN), "está" (ehs-TAH). Learning these patterns helps you sound more natural and confident, particularly important when working with elderly clients who may have hearing difficulties.

SPANISH GRAMMAR ESSENTIALS

Understanding basic Spanish grammar patterns is crucial for effective eldercare communication, as it allows you to create appropriate, respectful sentences rather than relying solely on memorized phrases. This section focuses on the most essential grammatical concepts you'll need when caring for Spanish-speaking elderly clients, emphasizing formal address patterns and the structures most commonly used in healthcare settings.

Formal Address - "Usted" vs "Tú"

The most critical grammatical concept in eldercare Spanish is the distinction between formal and informal address. Always use "usted" (formal "you") when speaking with elderly clients, regardless of how well you know them. This shows respect and acknowledges their dignity, which is paramount in Hispanic culture. "Usted" uses third-person verb forms: "¿Cómo está usted?" (How are you?), "¿Necesita usted ayuda?" (Do you need help?), "Usted debe tomar su medicina" (You should take your medicine).

When speaking about the elderly client to family members, use third-person forms: "Ella necesita descansar" (She needs to rest), "Él está mejor hoy" (He is better today). This grammatical pattern reinforces respectful communication throughout all eldercare interactions.

Essential Verb Conjugations

Focus on the most useful verbs in eldercare contexts, primarily in the present tense and formal command forms. "Estar" (to be - temporary states) is crucial for health status: "¿Cómo está?" (How are you?), "Estoy aquí para ayudarle" (I am here to help you), "¿Está cómodo?" (Are you comfortable?).

"Tener" (to have) is essential for expressing needs and symptoms: "¿Tiene dolor?" (Do you have pain?), "Tengo que tomar sus signos vitales" (I have to take your vital signs), "¿Tiene sed?" (Are you thirsty?). "Necesitar" (to need) and "querer" (to want) help identify client needs: "¿Necesita ir al baño?" (Do you need to go to the bathroom?), "¿Quiere más agua?" (Do you want more water?).

Question Formation

questions often begin with question words: "¿Cómo?" (How?), "¿Cuándo?" (When?), "¿Dónde?" (Where?), "¿Qué?" (What?). These combine with verbs to create essential eldercare questions: "¿Cómo se siente?" (How do you feel?), "¿Cuándo fue la última vez que comió?" (When did you last eat?), "¿Dónde le duele?" (Where does it hurt?).

Yes/no questions in Spanish can be formed by raising your voice at the end of a statement or by inverting word order: "¿Está cómodo?" (Are you comfortable?), "¿Necesita ayuda?" (Do you need help?). The upward intonation is particularly important when working with elderly clients who may have hearing difficulties.

Expressing Pain And Discomfort

Pain assessment requires specific grammatical structures. Use "doler" (to hurt) with indirect object pronouns: "Me duele la cabeza" (My head hurts), "¿Le duele aquí?" (Does this hurt you?), "¿Dónde le duele más?" (Where does it hurt you most?). The verb "sentir" (to feel) is useful for general discomfort: "¿Cómo se siente?" (How do you feel?), "Me siento mal" (I feel bad), "¿Se siente mejor?" (Do you feel better?).

Time Expressions

Learn basic time expressions: "por la mañana" (in the morning), "por la tarde" (in the afternoon), "por la noche" (at night), "antes de comer" (before eating), "después de cenar" (after dinner). Combine these with verbs: "Debe tomar su medicina por la mañana" (You should take your medicine in the morning), "Vamos a bañarle por la tarde" (We're going to bathe you in the afternoon).

Gentle Commands And Suggestions

When providing care instructions, use gentle, respectful command forms rather than harsh imperatives. Use "puede" (can) or "debe" (should) to soften requests: "Puede sentarse aquí" (You can sit here), "Debe beber más agua" (You should drink more water). The phrase "vamos a" (we're going to) creates a collaborative tone: "Vamos a revisar su presión" (We're going to check your blood pressure), "Vamos a cambiar su ropa" (We're going to change your clothes).

DAILY GREETINGS AND INTRODUCTIONS WITH ELDERLY PATIENTS

Key Vocabulary

Buenos días - BWEH-nos DEE-ahs - Good morning

Buenas tardes - BWEH-nahs TAHR-dehs - Good afternoon

¿Cómo está usted? - KOH-moh ehs-TAH oos-TEHD - How are you? (formal)

Mucho gusto - MOO-choh GOOS-toh - Nice to meet you

Me llamo... - meh YAH-moh - My name is...

¿Necesita algo? - neh-seh-SEE-tah AHL-goh - Do you need anything?

Voy a ayudarle - voy ah ah-yoo-DAHR-leh - I am going to help you

¿Tiene dolor? - TYEH-neh doh-LOHR - Are you in pain?

¿Listo para...? - LEES-toh PAH-rah - Ready for...?

Señora - seh-NYOH-rah - Ma'am / Mrs.

Señor - seh-NYOHR - Sir / Mr.

Gracias - GRAH-syahs - Thank you

Grammatical Examples

Buenos días, señor García. ¿Cómo está usted? - Good morning, Mr. Garcia. How are you?

Buenos días, señora López. ¿Cómo está usted? - Good morning, Mrs. Lopez. How are you?

Buenas tardes, señorita Ruiz. ¿Cómo está usted? - Good afternoon, Miss Ruiz. How are you?

Buenas noches, don Carlos. ¿Cómo está usted? - Good evening, Don Carlos. How are you?

Buenas noches, doña Carmen. ¿Cómo está usted? - Good evening, Doña Carmen. How are you?

Practice Dialog

Buenos días, señora. ¿Cómo amaneció hoy?

Buenos días, cariño. Muy bien, gracias a Dios. ¿Y usted cómo está?

Muy bien, gracias. ¿Le parece si primero revisamos sus signos vitales?

Por supuesto, no hay problema. Usted siempre es tan amable.

English translation:
Good morning, ma'am. How did you wake up today?

Good morning, dear. Very well, thank God. And how are you?

Very well, thank you. Would you mind if we check your vital signs first?

Of course, no problem. You are always so kind.

Practice Scenario

La auxiliar entra y sonríe. "Buenos días, señora García. Soy Elena, su ayudante hoy." La señora, confundida, la mira. "Voy a ayudarla a levantarse y vestirla para el desayuno." Elena habla claro y calmada, ofreciendo su brazo para apoyo. "¿Está lista?" La señora asiente lentamente, tomando el brazo con confianza para comenzar su rutina diaria.

English translation:
The aide enters and smiles. "Good morning, Mrs. Garcia. I am Elena, your helper today." The confused woman looks at her. "I am going to help you get up and dress for breakfast." Elena speaks clearly and calmly, offering her arm for support. "Are you ready?" The woman nods slowly, taking the arm with trust to begin their daily routine.

ASKING ABOUT COMFORT AND PAIN LEVELS

Key Vocabulary

¿Cómo se siente hoy? - KOH-moh seh see-EN-teh oy - How do you feel today?

¿Le duele algo? - leh doo-EH-leh AHL-goh - Are you in any pain?

¿Dónde le duele? - DOHN-deh leh doo-EH-leh - Where does it hurt?

¿Es un dolor fuerte? - ehs oon doh-LOHR FWEHR-teh - Is it a strong pain?

¿Se siente cómodo/a? - seh see-EN-teh KOH-moh-doh/dah - Are you comfortable?

Voy a ayudarle a moverse - voy ah ah-yoo-DAHR-leh ah moh-BEHR-seh - I am going to help you move

¿Necesita más almohadas? - neh-seh-SEE-tah mahs ahl-moh-AH-dahs - Do you need more pillows?

¿Le molesta la luz? - leh moh-LEHS-tah lah loos - Is the light bothering you?

¿Quiere que ajuste la cama? - kee-EH-reh keh ah-HOOS-teh lah KAH-mah - Would you like me to adjust the bed?

¿Le gustaría un masaje suave? - leh goos-tah-REE-ah oon mah-SAH-heh SWAH-beh - Would you like a gentle massage?

¿Está bien así? - ehs-TAH bee-ehn ah-SEE - Is this okay?

Avíseme si siente molestia - ah-BEE-seh-meh see see-EN-teh moh-LEHS-tyah - Let me know if you feel any discomfort

¿Se siente cómodo? - Do you feel comfortable? (formal, masculine)

¿Se siente cómoda? - Do you feel comfortable? (formal, feminine)

¿Te sientes cómodo? - Do you feel comfortable? (informal, masculine)

¿Te sientes cómoda? - Do you feel comfortable? (informal, feminine)

Practice Dialog

Buenos días, ¿cómo amaneció hoy? ¿Hay alguna molestia o dolor que deba saber?

Buenos días. La verdad, la espalda me duele un poco hoy, especialmente al moverme.

Entiendo. Voy a ayudarle a cambiar de posición para que esté más cómodo. ¿En una escala del uno al diez, cómo calificaría el dolor?

Diría que es un cuatro. Pero con un poco de ayuda, estoy seguro de que mejorará.

English translation:

Good morning, how are you feeling today? Is there any discomfort or pain I should know about?

Good morning. Truthfully, my back is hurting a bit today, especially when I move.

I understand. I am going to help you change positions so you are more comfortable. On a scale of one to ten, how would you rate the pain?

I would say it's a four. But with a little help, I'm sure it will get better.

Practice Scenario

La auxiliar Rosa pregunta: "Doña Carmen, ¿cómo está hoy? ¿Le duele la espalda o las articulaciones en una escala del uno al diez?" Doña Carmen responde con voz débil: "Un seis, hija". Rosa la ayuda a cambiar de posición en la cama, revisa la piel en busca de úlceras por presión y asegura que el colchón antiescaras esté correctamente colocado.

English translation:

The aide Rosa asks: "Doña Carmen, how are you today? Does your back or joints hurt on a scale of one to ten?" Doña Carmen replies in a weak voice: "A six, dear". Rosa helps her change position in bed, checks her skin for pressure ulcers, and ensures the anti-bedsore mattress is correctly placed.

EXPLAINING DAILY CARE ROUTINES

¿Necesita ayuda? - neh-seh-SEE-tah ah-YOO-dah - Do you need help?

Vamos a bañarnos - VAH-mohs ah bah-NYAR-nohs - Let's get you bathed

Es hora de su medicina - ehs OH-rah deh soo meh-dee-SEE-nah - It's time for your medicine

¿Tiene dolor? - TYEH-neh doh-LOHR - Are you in pain?

Voy a ayudarle a vestirse - voy ah ah-yoo-DAHR-leh ah vehs-TEER-seh - I am going to help you get dressed

¿Le gustaría comer? - leh goos-tah-REE-ah koh-MEHR - Would you like to eat?

Vamos a tomar una caminata - VAH-mohs ah toh-MAHR OO-nah kah-mee-NAH-tah - Let's go for a walk

Señor / Señora - seh-NYOHR / seh-NYOH-rah - Sir / Ma'am

¿Puede levantarse? - PWEH-deh leh-vahn-TAHR-seh - Can you get up?

Con cuidado - kohn kwee-DAH-doh - Carefully

¿Le aprieta el zapato? - leh ah-PRYEH-tah ehl sah-PAH-toh - Is the shoe too tight?

¿Le gustaría beber agua? - leh goos-tah-REE-ah beh-BEHR AH-gwah - Would you like to drink some water?

Grammatical Examples

Voy a ayudarle a bañarse ahora. - I am going to help you bathe now.

24

Voy a traerle el desayuno en cinco minutos. - I am going to bring you breakfast in five minutes.

Voy a tomarle la presión arterial. - I am going to take your blood pressure.

Voy a acompañarle a caminar. - I am going to accompany you for a walk.

Practice Dialog

Buenos días, ¿está listo para su baño? Vamos a usar agua tibia para que esté cómodo.

Sí, gracias. ¿Podemos cerrar la cortina un poco más? Hace algo de frío.

Por supuesto, así está mejor. Le voy a ayudar a lavarse el pelo con cuidado.

Eso se siente muy bien. Usted siempre es muy amable.

Practice Scenario

La auxiliar Rosa explica con calma la rutina a la Sra. Gómez. "Primero, el aseo personal en el baño con ayuda para la transferencia. Luego, revisamos sus signos vitales. Para la hidratación, tiene su botella de agua aquí. Más tarde, la movilizaremos para cambiar la ropa de cama y prevenir úlceras por presión. Su bienestar es nuestra prioridad."

English translation:

The aide Rosa calmly explains the routine to Mrs. Gómez. "First, personal hygiene in the bathroom with transfer assistance. Then, we check your vital signs. For hydration, your water bottle is here. Later, we will mobilize you to change the bed linens and prevent pressure ulcers. Your well-being is our priority."

BUILDING RAPPORT AND SHOWING RESPECT

Key Vocabulary

Buenos días - BWEH-nos DEE-as - Good morning

Buenas tardes - BWEH-nas TAR-des - Good afternoon

¿Cómo está usted? - KOH-moh ehs-TAH oos-TED - How are you? (formal)

Señor / Señora - seh-NYOR / seh-NYOR-ah - Sir / Ma'am

Por favor - por fah-VOR - Please

Gracias - GRAH-syahs - Thank you

Con permiso - kon per-MEE-so - Excuse me (to pass or enter)

¿Necesita ayuda? - neh-seh-SEE-tah ah-YOO-dah - Do you need help?

Así está bien - ah-SEE ehs-TAH byen - That's good, just like that

Descanse - des-KAN-seh - Rest

Estoy aquí para ayudarle - ehs-TOY ah-KEE pah-rah ah-yoo-DAR-leh - I am here to help you

Que se mejore - keh seh meh-HOR-eh - Get well soon

Grammatical Examples

¿Le gustaría un poco de agua? - Would you like some water?

¿Le gustaría un poco de té? - Would you like some tea?

¿Le gustaría escuchar música? - Would you like to listen to music?

¿Le gustaría que abriera la ventana? - Would you like me to open the window?

Buenos días, ¿cómo amaneció hoy?
Muy bien, gracias por preguntar. ¿Podría ayudarme a sentarme, por favor?
Por supuesto, tome su tiempo. Voy a ajustar las almohadas para que esté más cómoda.
Se lo agradezco mucho. Usted siempre es tan amable.

English translation:
Good morning, how are you feeling today?
Very well, thank you for asking. Could you help me sit up, please?
Of course, take your time. I'm going to adjust the pillows so you are more comfortable.
I appreciate that so much. You are always so kind.

Practice Scenario

La Sra. García, con demencia, se negaba al baño. Ana, su auxiliar, en lugar de insistir, le habló de su juventud. Le ofreció una toalla caliente y eligió su ropa favorita. Con paciencia y validando sus recuerdos, Ana ganó su confianza. La Sra. García accedió tranquilamente, sintiéndose escuchada y respetada en su rutina de cuidado personal.

English translation:
Mrs. Garcia, with dementia, refused her bath. Ana, her aide, instead of insisting, talked to her about her youth. She offered her a warm towel and chose her favorite clothes. With patience and validating her memories, Ana gained her trust. Mrs. Garcia agreed calmly, feeling heard and respected in her personal care routine.

COMMUNICATING WITH FAMILY MEMBERS

Buenos días - BWEH-nos DEE-as - Good morning

¿Cómo está? - KOH-moh ehs-TAH - How are you?

¿Necesita ayuda? - neh-seh-SEE-tah ah-YOO-dah - Do you need help?

Voy a ayudarle - voy ah ah-yoo-DAHR-leh - I am going to help you

Es hora de su medicina - ehs OH-rah deh soo meh-dee-SEE-nah - It is time for your medicine

¿Tiene dolor? - tee-EH-neh doh-LOHR - Do you have pain?

Vamos a comer - VAH-mos ah koh-MEHR - Let's eat

¿Quiere agua? - kee-EH-reh AH-gwah - Would you like some water?

Con cuidado - kohn kwee-DAH-doh - Carefully

Señor/Señora - seh-NYOR/seh-NYOR-ah - Sir/Madam

¿Le gustaría...? - leh goos-tah-REE-ah - Would you like...?

Descance - dehs-KAHN-seh - Rest

Grammatical Examples

¿Necesita usted ayuda para bañarse? - Do you need help bathing?

¿Necesita usted agua? - Do you need water?

¿Necesita usted que lea esta carta? - Do you need me to read this letter?

¿Necesita usted su medicina? - Do you need your medicine?

Practice Dialog

Buenos días, ¿cómo amaneció hoy? ¿Durmió bien?

Buenos días. Sí, gracias, descansé bien. ¿Podría ayudarme a sentarme, por favor?

Por supuesto, tome mi brazo. Vamos a levantarnos despacio para no marearse.

Muchas gracias, eres muy amable.

English translation:

Good morning, how did you wake up today? Did you sleep well?

Good morning. Yes, thank you, I rested well. Could you help me sit up, please?

Of course, take my arm. Let's get up slowly so you don't get dizzy.

Thank you very much, you are very kind.

Practice Scenario

La señora García, con demencia, repite las mismas preguntas. Su hija, frustrada, llama. La auxiliar de enfermería le sugiere: "Use frases cortas y reconfortantes". Al día siguiente, la hija dice: "Te quiero, mamá. Estás segura". La señora sonríe y susurra: "Mi niña". La comunicación afectiva es clave para el bienestar emocional del residente.

English translation: Mrs. Garcia, with dementia, repeats the same questions. Her daughter, frustrated, calls. The nursing assistant suggests: "Use short and comforting phrases." The next day, the daughter says: "I love you, mom. You are safe." Mrs. Garcia smiles and whispers: "My girl." Affective communication is key for the resident's emotional well-being.

ASSISTING WITH BATHING AND SHOWERING

¿Necesita ayuda para bañarse? - NEH-seh-see-tah ah-YOO-dah pah-rah bah-NYAR-seh - Do you need help bathing?

Vamos a ducharnos - VAH-mohs ah doo-CHAR-nohs - Let's take a shower.

¿Está listo/a? - ehs-TAH LEES-toh/tah - Are you ready?

Tenga cuidado - TEN-gah kwee-DAH-doh - Be careful.

Agua caliente - AH-gwah kah-lee-EN-teh - Hot water

Agua fría - AH-gwah FREE-ah - Cold water

Jabón - hah-BOHN - Soap

Champú - chahm-POO - Shampoo

Toalla - toh-AH-yah - Towel

¿Se siente mareado/a? - seh see-EN-teh mah-reh-AH-doh/dah - Do you feel dizzy?

Es hora de vestirse - ehs OH-rah deh vehs-TEER-seh - It's time to get dressed.

¿Está cómodo/a? - ehs-TAH KOH-moh-doh/dah - Are you comfortable?

Grammatical Examples

Voy a ayudarle con el baño. - I am going to help you with the bath.

Voy a ayudarle con la ducha. - I am going to help you with the shower.

Voy a ayudarle con la toalla. - I am going to help you with the towel.

Voy a ayudarle con el jabón. - I am going to help you with the soap.

Voy a ayudarle con el champú. - I am going to help you with the shampoo.

Voy a ayudarle con la bata. - I am going to help you with the robe.

Practice Dialog

Buenos días, ¿está listo para su baño? El agua está tibia, a una temperatura agradable.

Sí, gracias. Hoy me siento un poco débil, ¿me podría ayudar a entrar a la ducha?

Por supuesto, tómese de mi brazo. Voy a usar la silla para que esté más seguro.

Muy bien. Le agradezco mucho su paciencia y ayuda.

English translation:

Buenos días, ¿está listo para su baño? El agua está tibia, a una temperatura agradable.

Sí, gracias. Hoy me siento un poco débil, ¿me podría ayudar a entrar a la ducha?

Por supuesto, tómese de mi brazo. Voy a usar la silla para que esté más seguro.

Muy bien. Le agradezco mucho su paciencia y ayuda.

Practice Scenario

La señora García permite que la auxiliar le ayude con la ducha. La auxiliar verifica la temperatura del agua y usa un banco de ducha para mayor seguridad. Con guantes, lava suavemente la espalda de la señora con jabón suave. Le seca con una toalla suave y aplica loción en su piel frágil. La auxiliar la viste con una bata limpia, asegurando su dignidad en todo momento.

English translation: Mrs. García allows the aide to help her with the shower. The aide checks the water temperature and uses a shower chair for safety. With gloves, she gently washes the señora's back with mild soap. She dries her with a soft towel and applies lotion to her fragile skin. The aide dresses her in a clean robe, ensuring her dignity at all times.

HELP WITH DRESSING AND GROOMING

¿Le ayudo a vestirse? - ah-YOO-doh ah vehs-TEER-seh - May I help you get dressed?

Vamos a ponernos la camisa - VAH-mohs ah poh-NEHR-nohs lah kah-MEE-sah - Let's put on our shirt

Levante el brazo, por favor - leh-VAHN-teh ehl BRAH-soh pohr fah-VOHR - Lift your arm, please

¿Está cómodo/a? - ehs-TAH KOH-moh-doh/dah - Are you comfortable?

Vamos a peinarnos - VAH-mohs ah pay-NAHR-nohs - Let's comb our hair

Abrochemos los botones - ah-broh-CHEH-mohs lohs boh-TOH-nehs - Let's button the buttons

¿Puede inclinarse hacia adelante? - PWEH-deh een-klee-NAHR-seh AH-see-ah ah-deh-LAHN-teh - Can you lean forward?

Voy a ayudarle con los zapatos - voy ah ah-yoo-DAHR-leh kohn lohs sah-PAH-tohs - I am going to help you with your shoes

¿Necesita usar el baño? - neh-seh-SEE-tah oo-SAHR ehl BAH-nyoh - Do you need to use the bathroom?

Vamos a lavarnos la cara - VAH-mohs ah lah-VAHR-nohs lah KAH-rah - Let's wash our face

Tome mi brazo - TOH-meh mee BRAH-soh - Take my arm

¿Le duele algo? - leh DWEH-leh AHL-goh - Is anything hurting you?

Voy a ayudarle a ponerse la camisa. - I am going to help you put on your shirt.

Voy a ayudarle a peinarse. - I am going to help you comb your hair.

Voy a ayudarle a lavarse la cara. - I am going to help you wash your face.

Voy a ayudarle a afeitarse. - I am going to help you shave.

Voy a ayudarle a atarse los zapatos. - I am going to help you tie your shoes.

Practice Dialog

Buenos días, ¿está listo para vestirse? Hoy hace fresco, le preparé su suéter azul.

Sí, por favor. ¿Me podría ayudar a abrochar los botones? Las manos no me responden como antes.

Claro que sí, no se preocupe. Voy a ayudarle con los botones y luego a peinarlo suavemente.

Muchas gracias. Se siente uno mucho mejor cuando está arregladito.

English translation:

Good morning, are you ready to get dressed? It's cool today, I prepared your blue sweater.

Yes, please. Could you help me button the buttons? My hands don't work like they used to.

Of course, don't worry. I will help you with the buttons and then gently comb your hair.

Thank you very much. One feels so much better when they are nicely groomed.

Practice Scenario

La señora Rosa permite que la auxiliar le ayude a vestirse. Juntas eligen un vestido cómodo. La auxiliar le ayuda con la higiene bucal y a peinarse, explicando cada paso con paciencia. Rosa sonríe al verse en el espejo, sintiéndose arreglada y respetada. La rutina diaria de cuidado refuerza su dignidad y bienestar.

English translation: Mrs. Rosa allows the aide to help her get dressed. Together they choose a comfortable dress. The aide helps with her oral hygiene and to comb her hair, explaining each step patiently. Rosa smiles seeing herself in the mirror, feeling groomed and respected. The daily care routine reinforces her dignity and well-being.

ORAL CARE AND DENTAL HYGIENE

Buenos días - BWEH-nos DEE-as - Good morning

Vamos a limpiar los dientes - VAH-mos ah leem-pee-AR lohs dee-EN-tes - We are going to clean your teeth

Por favor, abra la boca - por fah-VOR, AH-brah lah BOH-kah - Please open your mouth

Necesito revisar su dentadura postiza - neh-seh-SEE-toh reh-bee-SAR soo den-tah-DOO-rah pos-TEE-sah - I need to check your dentures

¿Le duele alguna muela? - leh DOO-eh-leh ahl-GOO-nah MWEH-lah - Does any tooth hurt?

Voy a cepillar suavemente - voy ah seh-pee-YAR swah-veh-MEN-teh - I am going to brush gently

Vamos a enjuagar - VAH-mos ah en-wah-GAR - Let's rinse

¿Tiene sensibilidad? - tee-EN-eh sen-see-bee-lee-DAD - Do you have sensitivity?

Aquí tiene el vaso para escupir - ah-KEE tee-EN-eh el VAH-so PAH-rah es-koo-PEER - Here is the cup to spit

Sus prótesis están limpias - soos PRO-teh-sis es-TAN LEEM-pee-as - Your dentures are clean

¿Se siente cómodo/a? - seh see-EN-teh KOH-moh-doh/dah - Are you comfortable?

Gracias por su cooperación - GRAH-see-as por soo koh-op-eh-rah-see-ON - Thank you for your cooperation

Vamos a cepillar los dientes suavemente. - We are going to brush the teeth gently.

Vamos a limpiar la dentadura postiza con cuidado. - We are going to clean the dentures carefully.

Vamos a usar el hilo dental con paciencia. - We are going to use the dental floss patiently.

Vamos a enjuagar la boca completamente. - We are going to rinse the mouth completely.

Practice Dialog

Buenos días. ¿Está listo para cepillarse los dientes? Le tengo su cepillo suave y pasta dental con flúor.

Sí, gracias. ¿Podría ayudarme un poco hoy? Mis manos no están muy fuertes.

Por supuesto. Cepillaremos suavemente para limpiar bien todas las piezas dentales y cuidar sus encías.

Muy bien. Después me gustaría usar el enjuague bucal sin alcohol para sentirme más fresca.

English translation:

Good morning. Are you ready to brush your teeth? I have your soft toothbrush and fluoride toothpaste.

Yes, thank you. Could you help me a little today? My hands aren't very strong.

Of course. We will brush gently to clean all your teeth well and take care of your gums.

Very good. Afterward, I would like to use the alcohol-free mouthwash to feel fresher.

Practice Scenario

La señora García se resiste al cuidado bucal. Su cuidadora, Elena, habla con calma. "Abra la boca, por favor". Usa un cepillo suave y pasta dental. Elena limpia suavemente las encías y la dentadura postiza, revisando si hay llagas. "Muy bien, señora". Una sonrisa breve aparece. La higiene oral diaria previene infecciones y mantiene su comodidad y dignidad.

English translation:

Mrs. García resists oral care. Her caregiver, Elena, speaks calmly. "Open your mouth, please". She uses a soft brush and toothpaste. Elena gently cleans the gums and dentures, checking for sores. "Very good, ma'am". A brief smile appears. Daily oral hygiene prevents infections and maintains her comfort and dignity.

TOILETING ASSISTANCE AND INCONTINENCE CARE

¿Necesita usar el baño? - neh-seh-SEE-tah oo-SAHR ehl BAH-nyoh - Do you need to use the bathroom?

Vamos al baño - VAH-mohs ahl BAH-nyoh - Let's go to the bathroom

Pañal - pah-NYAHL - Diaper

Necesito cambiarle el pañal - neh-seh-SEE-toh kahm-bee-AHR-leh ehl pah-NYAHL - I need to change your diaper

Voy a ayudarle a limpiarse - voy ah ah-yoo-DAHR-leh ah leem-pee-AHR-seh - I am going to help you clean yourself

¿Se siente limpio y seco? - seh see-EN-teh LEEM-pee-oh ee SEH-koh - Do you feel clean and dry?

Vamos a lavarnos las manos - VAH-mohs ah lah-VAHR-nohs lahs MAH-nohs - Let's wash our hands

Protector de cama - proh-tek-TOHR deh KAH-mah - Bed protector

Orina - oh-REE-nah - Urine

Deposición - deh-poh-see-see-OHN - Bowel movement

¿Tiene alguna molestia? - tee-EH-neh ahl-GOO-nah moh-LEHS-tee-ah - Do you have any discomfort?

¿Le duele algo? - leh doo-EH-leh AHL-goh - Does anything hurt?

Grammatical Examples

Voy a ayudarle a ir al baño. - I am going to help you go to the bathroom.

Voy a traerle una toalla limpia. - I am going to bring you a clean towel.

Voy a cambiarle la sábana ahora. - I am going to change your sheet now.

Voy a buscar el carro de la ducha. - I am going to get the shower chair.

Voy a prepararle el baño. - I am going to prepare your bath for you.

Practice Dialog

¿Señora, necesita ayuda para ir al baño o prefiere que le traiga la cuña?

Creo que sería mejor la cuña, por favor. No me siento muy segura para caminar.

Claro, enseguida se la traigo. Después, la ayudaré a limpiarse y a cambiarse para que esté más cómoda.

Muchas gracias, cariño. Disculpe las molestias.

English translation:

Ma'am, do you need help going to the bathroom, or would you prefer I bring you the bedpan?

I think the bedpan would be better, please. I don't feel very steady to walk.

Of course, I'll bring it right away. Afterwards, I will help you clean up and get changed so you are more comfortable.

Thank you very much, dear. Sorry for the trouble.

Practice Scenario

La señora García mojó la cama. Su auxiliar de enfermería, Elena, la ayudó a levantarse con suavidad. "No se preocupe, es común", dijo tranquilamente mientras la llevaba al baño. Le proporcionó cuidado perineal, la secó y le puso ropa limpia y una braga absorbente nueva. Mantuvieron su dignidad con cada gesto, asegurando su comodidad e higiene.

English translation: Mrs. Garcia wet the bed. Her nursing

assistant, Elena, helped her up gently. "Don't worry, it's common," she said calmly while taking her to the bathroom. She provided perineal care, dried her, and put on clean clothes and a new absorbent brief. They maintained her dignity with every gesture, ensuring her comfort and hygiene.

SKIN CARE AND PREVENTING BED SORES

¿Necesita ayuda para moverse? - neh-seh-SEE-tah ah-YOO-dah pah-rah moh-BEHR-seh - Do you need help moving?

Vamos a cambiar de posición - VAH-mohs ah kahm-bee-AHR deh poh-see-see-OHN - We are going to change your position

Voy a revisar su piel - voy ah reh-vee-SAHR soo pee-EL - I am going to check your skin

Mantengamos la piel limpia y seca - mahn-ten-GAH-mohs lah pee-EL LEEM-pee-ah ee SEH-kah - Let's keep the skin clean and dry

¿Le duele aquí? - leh doo-EH-leh ah-KEE - Does it hurt here?

Voy a aplicar crema hidratante - voy ah ah-plee-KAHR KREH-mah ee-drah-TAHN-teh - I am going to apply moisturizing cream

Es importante moverse - ehs eem-pohr-TAHN-teh moh-BEHR-seh - It is important to move

Usemos una almohada para apoyarle - oo-SEH-mohs OO-nah ahl-moh-AH-dah pah-rah ah-poy-AHR-leh - Let's use a pillow to support you

¿Se siente cómodo/a? - seh see-EN-teh KOH-moh-doh/dah - Are you comfortable?

Vamos a bañarle - VAH-mohs ah bah-NYAHR-leh - We are going to bathe you

¿Tiene comezón o ardor? - tee-EH-neh koh-meh-SOHN oh ahr-

DOHR - Do you have itching or burning?
Señor/Señora - seh-NYOHR/seh-NYOH-rah - Sir/Ma'am

Grammatical Examples

La piel está limpia. - The skin is clean.
La crema es suave. - The cream is soft.
La herida es profunda. - The wound is deep.
La almohada es cómoda. - The pillow is comfortable.
La paciente es tranquila. - The patient is calm.
La toalla está seca. - The towel is dry.

Practice Dialog

Vamos a girarlo suavemente para proteger su piel y mejorar la circulación.
Sí, y después aplicaremos la crema hidratante en la espalda para prevenir rozaduras.
¿La crema con óxido de zinc que usamos ayer?
Exactamente, esa misma. Es muy efectiva para mantener la piel sana y evitar úlceras.

English translation:
Let's turn you gently to protect your skin and improve circulation.
Yes, and then we'll apply the moisturizing cream to your back to prevent chafing.
The zinc oxide cream we used yesterday?
Exactly, that one. It's very effective for keeping the skin healthy and preventing bed sores.

Practice Scenario

La auxiliar Marta gira suavemente a doña Carmen para prevenir úlceras por presión. Limpia la piel con un limpiador suave, aplica crema barrera y seca bien las zonas de riesgo. Coloca una almohada entre sus rodillas para aliviar la presión. "Su piel se ve muy bien hoy", dice Marta con una sonrisa, asegurando su comodidad con un cuidado preventivo y respetuoso.

English translation:
The aide Marta gently turns Doña Carmen to prevent pressure ulcers. She cleans the skin with a gentle cleanser, applies barrier cream, and dries the risk areas well. She places a pillow between her knees to relieve pressure. "Your skin looks very good today," says Marta with a smile, ensuring her comfort with preventive and respectful care.

HELPING WITH WALKING AND TRANSFERS

Key Vocabulary

¿Le gustaría pararse? - leh goos-tah-REE-ah pah-RAHR-seh - Would you like to stand up?

Vamos a caminar un poco - VAH-mohs ah kah-mee-NAHR oon POH-koh - Let's walk a little bit.

Tome mi brazo - TOH-meh mee BRAH-soh - Take my arm.

Despacio - dehs-PAH-see-oh - Slowly.

Siéntese aquí, por favor - see-EN-teh-seh ah-KEE pohr fah-VOHR - Sit down here, please.

Con cuidado - kohn kwee-DAH-doh - Carefully.

¿Necesita descansar? - neh-seh-SEE-tah dehs-kahn-SAHR - Do you need to rest?

Le ayudo a levantarse - leh ah-YOO-doh ah leh-vahn-TAHR-seh - I will help you get up.

Apóyese en mí - ah-POH-yeh-seh ehn MEE - Lean on me.

Un paso a la vez - oon PAH-soh ah lah vehs - One step at a time.

¿Se siente mareado/a? - seh see-EN-teh mah-reh-AH-doh/dah - Do you feel dizzy?

Agárrese fuerte - ah-GAH-reh-seh FWEHR-teh - Hold on tight.

Grammatical Examples

Voy a ayudarle a caminar. - I am going to help you (formal) to walk.

Voy a ayudarle a pararse. - I am going to help you (formal) to stand up.

Voy a ayudarle a sentarse. - I am going to help you (formal) to sit down.

Voy a ayudarle a transferirse. - I am going to help you (formal) to transfer.

Vamos a levantarnos despacio. ¿Está listo?

Sí, estoy listo. Agárrame del brazo, por favor.

Perfecto. Uno, dos, tres... ¡Ahí está! Muy bien.

Gracias por su paciencia. Me siento más seguro con su ayuda.

English translation:

Let's stand up slowly. Are you ready?

Yes, I'm ready. Hold my arm, please.

Perfect. One, two, three... There we go! Very good.

Thank you for your patience. I feel safer with your help.

La Sra. García se levanta lentamente de la cama con ayuda. La auxiliar le coloca el cinturón de soporte para transferirla de manera segura al sillón. "Paso a paso, señora, yo la ayudo", dice con calma. Usan el andador para ir al comedor, priorizando su seguridad y autonomía en cada movimiento con paciencia y respeto.

English translation:

Mrs. Garcia gets out of bed slowly with help. The aide places the gait belt to safely transfer her to the armchair. "Step by step, ma'am, I'll help you", she says calmly. They use the walker to go to the dining room, prioritizing her safety and autonomy in each movement with patience and respect.

USING WHEELCHAIRS AND MOBILITY AIDS

Key Vocabulary

¿Necesita ayuda para moverse? - neh-seh-SEE-tah ah-YOO-dah PAH-rah moh-VEHR-seh - Do you need help moving?

Vamos a sentarnos - VAH-mohs ah sen-TAHR-nohs - Let's sit down

¿Le duele aquí? - leh doo-EH-leh ah-KEE - Does it hurt here?

Vamos a usar la silla de ruedas - VAH-mohs ah oo-SAHR lah SEE-yah deh RWEH-dahs - We are going to use the wheelchair

¿Está cómodo/a? - ehs-TAH KOH-moh-doh/dah - Are you comfortable?

Con cuidado - kohn kwee-DAH-doh - Carefully

Agarre mi brazo - ah-GAH-rreh mee BRAH-soh - Hold my arm

Vamos a pararnos lentamente - VAH-mohs ah pah-RAHR-nohs len-tah-MEN-teh - Let's stand up slowly

¿Puede empujar la rueda? - PWEH-deh em-poo-HAHR lah RWEH-dah - Can you push the wheel?

Buenos días, señor/señora - BWEH-nohs DEE-ahs, seh-NYOHR/seh-NYOH-rah - Good morning, sir/ma'am

¿Le ajusto el cojín? - leh ah-HOO-stoh el koh-HEEN - Shall I adjust your cushion?

¿Listo/a para pasear? - LEES-toh/tah PAH-rah pah-seh-AHR - Ready for a walk?

Grammatical Examples

Voy a empujar su silla de ruedas con cuidado. - I am going to push your wheelchair carefully.

Vamos a empujar su silla de ruedas con cuidado. - We are going to push your wheelchair carefully.

Él va a empujar su silla de ruedas con cuidado. - He is going to push your wheelchair carefully.

Ella va a empujar su silla de ruedas con cuidado. - She is going to push your wheelchair carefully.

Practice Dialog

¿Le gustaría que ajustemos el respaldo de su silla para que esté más cómodo?

Sí, por favor. Así podré descansar mejor la espalda.

Perfecto. Ahora voy a asegurar los frenos antes de ayudarle a levantarse.

Gracias, así me siento mucho más segura.

English translation:

Would you like us to adjust the back of your chair so you're more comfortable?

Yes, please. That way I can rest my back better.

Perfect. Now I'm going to secure the brakes before helping you up.

Thank you, that makes me feel much safer.

Practice Scenario

La Sra. García, usuaria de silla de ruedas, se resiste a la transferencia. La auxiliar, Ana, explica cada paso con calma. "Voy a bloquear las ruedas y usar la cincha de transferencia para mayor seguridad". La Sra. García colabora. Después, Ana verifica la alineación postural y coloca los cojines de apoyo, asegurando su comodidad y prevención de úlceras por presión.

English translation:

Mrs. Garcia, a wheelchair user, resists the transfer. The aide, Ana, explains each step calmly. "I will lock the wheels and use the transfer belt for safety." Mrs. Garcia cooperates. Afterwards, Ana checks her postural alignment and places support cushions, ensuring her comfort and preventing pressure ulcers.

FALL PREVENTION
AND SAFETY

¿Necesita ayuda? - neh-seh-SEE-tah ah-YOO-dah - Do you need help?

Tome mi brazo - TOH-meh mee BRAH-soh - Take my arm

Vamos despacio - VAH-mohs des-PAH-syoh - Let's go slowly

¿Se siente mareado/a? - seh see-EN-teh mah-reh-AH-doh/dah - Do you feel dizzy?

El piso está resbaloso - ehl PEE-soh ehs-TAH res-bah-LOH-soh - The floor is slippery

Tenga cuidado - TEN-gah kwee-DAH-doh - Be careful

Use el pasamanos - OO-seh ehl pah-sah-MAH-nohs - Use the handrail

Siéntese, por favor - see-EN-teh-seh pohr fah-VOHR - Please sit down

Levántese lentamente - leh-VAHN-teh-seh len-tah-MEN-teh - Stand up slowly

Sus zapatos - soos sah-PAH-tohs - Your shoes

¿Puede pararse? - PWEH-deh pah-RAHR-seh - Can you stand up?

¿Hay algo en el camino? - aye AHL-goh en ehl kah-MEE-noh - Is there anything in your path?

Asegúrese de que el pasillo esté despejado. - Make sure the hallway is clear.

Asegúrese de que la habitación esté ordenada. - Make sure the bedroom is tidy.

Asegúrese de que el suelo esté seco. - Make sure the floor is dry.
Asegúrese de que las zapatillas estén bien ajustadas. - Make sure the slippers are well-fitted.

Practice Dialog

Recuerde, si necesita levantarse, por favor llámeme primero para que la ayude.

Tiene razón, no debo intentarlo solo. ¿Podría revisar que mi andador esté cerca?

Por supuesto, aquí está. Y recuerde usar siempre sus zapatos antideslizantes.

Gracias. Me siento más seguro con su ayuda y siguiendo estos consejos.

English translation:
Remember, if you need to get up, please call me first so I can help you.

You're right, I shouldn't try it alone. Could you check that my walker is close by?

Of course, here it is. And remember to always wear your non-slip shoes.

Thank you. I feel safer with your help and by following this advice.

Practice Scenario

La Sra. García se levantó rápidamente de la cama. "¡Tranquila, voy a ayudarla!", dijo la auxiliar de enfermería, acercándose. Le recordó usar su andador. Juntas revisaron que las luces estuvieran encendidas y que no hubiera obstáculos en el suelo. La Sra. García agradeció el apoyo de su brazo mientras caminaban con seguridad al comedor.

English translation:
Mrs. Garcia got out of bed quickly. "Easy, I will help you!", said the nurse aide, approaching. She reminded her to use her walker. Together they checked that the lights were on and that there were no obstacles on the floor. Mrs. Garcia thanked her for the

support of her arm as they walked safely to the dining room.

POSITIONING IN BED AND TURNING PATIENTS

Voy a ayudarle a moverse - voy ah ah-yoo-DAR-leh ah moh-BEHR-seh - I am going to help you move

Vamos a girar hacia su lado - VAH-mohs ah hee-RAR ah-see-ah soo LAH-doh - Let's turn to your side

¿Puede doblar las rodillas? - PWEH-deh doh-BLAR lahs roh-DEE-yahs - Can you bend your knees?

Levántese un poco - leh-VAHN-teh-seh oon POH-koh - Lift up a little

Apóyese en mí - ah-POH-yeh-seh ehn mee - Lean on me

¿Está cómodo/a? - ehs-TAH KOH-moh-doh/dah - Are you comfortable?

Voy a ajustar su almohada - voy ah ah-hoos-TAR soo ahl-moh-AH-dah - I am going to adjust your pillow

Necesita cambiar de posición - neh-seh-SEE-tah kahm-bee-AR deh poh-see-see-OHN - You need to change position

Use mis hombros para empujar - OO-seh mees OHM-brohs PAH-rah ehm-poo-HAR - Use my shoulders to push

Deslícese hacia mí - dehs-LEE-eh-seh ah-see-ah mee - Slide towards me

Voy a poner una cuña - voy ah poh-NEHR OO-nah KOO-nyah - I am going to place a pillow/wedge

¿Le duele algo en esta posición? - leh DWEH-leh AHL-goh ehn

EHS-tah poh-see-see-OHN - Does anything hurt in this position?

Grammatical Examples

Vamos a girar al señor hacia su lado derecho. - We are going to turn the gentleman onto his right side.

Vamos a girar a la señora hacia su lado izquierdo. - We are going to turn the lady onto her left side.

Vamos a girar al paciente hacia su lado derecho. - We are going to turn the male patient onto his right side.

Vamos a girar a la paciente hacia su lado izquierdo. - We are going to turn the female patient onto her left side.

Practice Dialog

Voy a ayudarle a girarse hacia su lado izquierdo. ¿Está listo?
Sí, estoy listo. ¿Debo agarrarme de la baranda?
Así es, sujétese firme. Uno, dos, tres... ¡allá vamos!
Gracias, así estoy mucho más cómodo.

English translation:
I'm going to help you turn onto your left side. Are you ready?
Yes, I'm ready. Should I hold onto the rail?
That's right, hold on tight. One, two, three... here we go!
Thank you, this is much more comfortable.

Practice Scenario

La auxiliar Marta coloca la almohada de cuña para mantener a la señora Elena de lado, previniendo úlceras por presión. Levanta la baranda de seguridad y verifica que esté cómoda. "¿Necesita algo más?", pregunta suavemente. Elena niega con la cabeza, sonriendo. Marta documenta los cambios en la piel y el repositioning en el informe de cuidados.

English translation:
The aide Marta places the wedge pillow to keep Mrs. Elena on her side, preventing pressure ulcers. She raises the safety rail and verifies she is comfortable. "Do you need anything else?", she asks softly. Elena shakes her head, smiling. Marta documents the

skin changes and the repositioning in the care report.

PHYSICAL THERAPY EXERCISES AND ENCOURAGEMENT

Key Vocabulary

Vamos a caminar un poco - VAH-mohs ah kah-mee-NAHR oon POH-koh - Let's walk a little

Respire profundamente - rehs-PEE-reh proh-foon-dah-MEN-teh - Breathe deeply

Muy bien - MOO-ee bee-EN - Very good

¿Le duele aquí? - Leh doo-EH-leh ah-KEE - Does it hurt here?

Necesito que se siente, por favor - Neh-seh-SEE-toh keh seh see-EN-teh, pohr fah-VOHR - I need you to sit down, please

Un paso a la vez - Oon PAH-soh ah lah vehs - One step at a time

Vamos a estirar la pierna - VAH-mohs ah ehs-tee-RAHR lah pee-EHR-nah - Let's stretch your leg

Descanse un momento - dehs-KAHN-seh oon moh-MEN-toh - Rest a moment

Por aquí, señora/señor - Pohr ah-KEE, seh-NYOH-rah/seh-NYOHR - This way, ma'am/sir

Tranquilo/a - trahn-KEE-loh/lah - Relax, stay calm

¿Puede pararse? - PWEH-deh pah-RAHR-seh - Can you stand up?

Agárrese de mi brazo - ah-GAH-reh-seh deh mee BRAH-soh - Hold onto my arm

Grammatical Examples

Ahora levante el brazo derecho. - Now raise your right arm.

Ahora levante la pierna derecha. - Now raise your right leg.

Ahora levante el brazo izquierdo. - Now raise your left arm.
Ahora levante la pierna izquierda. - Now raise your left leg.

Practice Dialog

Muy bien, hoy vamos a hacer diez repeticiones con cada pierna.
Está bien, lo intentaré, pero me canso muy rápido.
Usted lo está haciendo excelente. Recuerde que cada pequeño esfuerzo cuenta.
Gracias por su paciencia. Me siento más fuerte cada día.

English translation:
Very good, today we are going to do ten repetitions with each leg.
Okay, I will try, but I get tired very quickly.
You are doing excellently. Remember that every little effort counts.
Thank you for your patience. I feel stronger every day.

Practice Scenario

La señora Rosa realiza sus ejercicios de terapia física con su auxiliar. Con paciencia, el auxiliar le guía en las flexiones de rodillas y los levantamientos de brazo. "Respire hondo, usted puede", la anima suavemente. Cada pequeño movimiento fortalece sus músculos y mejora su movilidad, clave para mantener su independencia en el hogar de ancianos.

English translation: Mrs. Rosa does her physical therapy exercises with her aide. With patience, the aide guides her through knee bends and arm raises. "Breathe deeply, you can do it," he encourages softly. Each small movement strengthens her muscles and improves her mobility, key to maintaining her independence in the nursing home.

MEDICATION REMINDERS AND ADMINISTRATION

Key Vocabulary

¿Necesita tomar su medicina ahora? - neh-seh-SEE-tah toh-MAHR soo meh-dee-SEE-nah ah-OH-rah - Do you need to take your medicine now?

Con comida - kohn koh-MEE-dah - With food

Con agua - kohn AH-gwah - With water

Abra la boca, por favor - AH-brah lah BOH-kah pohr fah-VOHR - Open your mouth, please

Trague, por favor - TRAH-geh pohr fah-VOHR - Swallow, please

¿Le duele algo? - leh doo-EH-leh AHL-goh - Are you in any pain?

Es hora de sus pastillas - ehs OH-rah deh soos pahs-TEE-yahs - It's time for your pills

Voy a tomar su presión arterial - voy ah toh-MAHR soo preh-see-OHN ahr-teh-ree-AHL - I am going to take your blood pressure

¿Tiene alergias a algún medicamento? - tee-EH-neh ah-LEHR-hee-ahs ah ahl-GOON meh-dee-kah-MEN-toh - Do you have allergies to any medication?

¿Puede sentarse derecho para tragar? - PWEH-deh sen-TAHR-seh deh-REH-choh PAH-rah trah-GAHR - Can you sit up straight to swallow?

Vamos a revisar sus medicamentos - VAH-mohs ah reh-bee-SAHR soos meh-dee-kah-MEN-tohs - Let's review your medications

¿Tiene dificultad para tragar? - tee-EH-neh dee-fee-kool-TAHD PAH-rah trah-GAHR - Do you have difficulty swallowing?

Grammatical Examples

Es hora de su medicamento. - It is time for your medication.
Es hora de su chequeo. - It is time for your check-up.
Es hora de su cita. - It is time for your appointment.
Es hora de su descanso. - It is time for your rest.

Practice Dialog

Buenos días, es hora de su medicamento para la presión arterial. Aquí tiene un vaso de agua.
Sí, gracias. ¿Son las pastillas blancas las que debo tomar con el desayuno?
Así es. Solo necesita tomar una. ¿Le puedo ayudar con algo más?
No, está bien. Me las tomo y luego vamos a desayunar.

English translation:
Good morning, it's time for your blood pressure medication. Here's a glass of water.
Yes, thank you. Are the white pills the ones I take with breakfast?
That's right. You only need to take one. Can I help you with anything else?
No, it's fine. I'll take them and then we'll have breakfast.

Practice Scenario

La enfermera Carmen revisa el cartón de pastillas. "Señora Luisa, es hora de su medicamento para la presión", dice suavemente. Observa mientras Luisa traga la pastilla con agua. Carmen registra la dosis en la hoja de administración, asegurándose de la hora y la medicación correcta. Le sonríe. "Muy bien, hasta la próxima dosis". Su supervisión meticulosa garantiza seguridad.

English translation:
Nurse Carmen checks the pill organizer. "Mrs. Luisa, it's time for your blood pressure medication," she says softly. She watches as Luisa swallows the pill with water. Carmen records the dose

on the medication administration record, ensuring the correct time and medication. She smiles. "Very good, see you at the next dose." Her meticulous oversight ensures safety.

EXPLAINING PILL SCHEDULES

¿Toma sus medicamentos? - TOH-mah soos meh-dee-kah-MEN-tohs - Do you take your medications?

Es hora de su medicina - ehs OH-rah deh soo meh-dee-SEE-nah - It's time for your medicine

Con comida - kohn koh-MEE-dah - With food

Con el estómago vacío - kohn ehl ehs-TOH-mah-goh vah-SEE-oh - On an empty stomach

Una vez al día - OO-nah vehs ahl DEE-ah - Once a day

Dos veces al día - dohs VEH-sehs ahl DEE-ah - Twice a day

Tome esto con agua - TOH-meh EHS-toh kohn AH-gwah - Take this with water

¿Tiene alguna alergia? - tee-EH-neh ahl-GOO-nah ah-LEHR-hee-ah - Do you have any allergies?

¿Le duele el estómago? - leh doo-EH-leh ehl ehs-TOH-mah-goh - Does your stomach hurt?

¿Necesita ayuda? - neh-seh-SEE-tah ah-YOO-dah - Do you need help?

Por favor, abra la boca - pohr fah-BOHR, AH-brah lah BOH-kah - Please, open your mouth

Que se mejore pronto - keh seh meh-HOH-reh PROHN-toh - Get well soon

Grammatical Examples

Usted toma la pastilla a las ocho de la mañana. - You take the pill at eight in the morning.

Usted toma la pastilla con el desayuno. - You take the pill with breakfast.

Usted toma la pastilla con un vaso de agua. - You take the pill with a glass of water.

Usted toma la pastilla antes de acostarse. - You take the pill before going to bed.

Practice Dialog

Ya tomó la pastilla para la presión, ahora le toca la de las ocho con la comida.

Perfecto, voy a anotarlo en el registro. ¿Necesita ayuda para tomar agua?

Sí, por favor. ¿La de color rosado también es para ahora?

No, esa es para después de cenar. Se la daremos más tarde.

Practice Scenario

La enfermera explica el horario de medicamentos a la nueva residente. "Señora García, tome la pastilla azul para la presión arterial con el desayuno. La tableta blanca, para el dolor, es según sea necesario después del almuerzo. Revisaré con usted más tarde". La señora García asiente, agradecida por la paciencia y la claridad.

English translation:

The nurse explains the medication schedule to the new resident. "Mrs. Garcia, take the blue pill for your blood pressure with breakfast. The white tablet, for pain, is as needed after lunch. I will check back with you later." Mrs. Garcia nods, grateful for the patience and clarity.

REPORTING SIDE EFFECTS OR CONCERNS

Key Vocabulary

¿Cómo se siente hoy? - KOH-moh seh SYEN-teh oy - How do you feel today?

¿Tiene algún dolor? - TYEH-neh ahl-GOON doh-LOHR - Do you have any pain?

¿Le duele aquí? - Leh DWEH-leh ah-KEE - Does it hurt here?

Señor/Señora - seh-NYOR / seh-NYOR-ah - Sir/Ma'am

¿Tuvo náuseas? - TOO-boh NOW-seh-ahs - Did you have nausea?

¿Se cayó? - seh kah-YOH - Did you fall?

Está mareado/mareada - eh-STAH mah-reh-AH-doh / mah-reh-AH-dah - You are dizzy

¿Puede describir la molestia? - PWEH-deh des-kree-BEER lah moh-LES-tyah - Can you describe the discomfort?

¿Cómo está su apetito? - KOH-moh eh-STAH soo ah-peh-TEE-toh - How is your appetite?

Está confundido/confundida - eh-STAH kohn-foon-DEE-doh / kohn-foon-DEE-dah - You are confused

¿Tuvo problemas para dormir? - TOO-boh proh-BLEH-mahs PAH-rah dor-MEER - Did you have trouble sleeping?

Revisar sus signos vitales - reh-bee-SAHR soos SEEG-nohs vee-TAH-les - To check your vital signs

Grammatical Examples

El señor parece confundido. - The gentleman seems confused.

62

La señora parece confundida. - The lady seems confused.
El paciente parece débil. - The patient (male) seems weak.
La paciente parece débil. - The patient (female) seems weak.
La medicina parece fuerte. - The medicine seems strong.
La situación parece seria. - The situation seems serious.

Practice Dialog

He notado que ha estado más somnoliento desde que empezó el nuevo medicamento.
Sí, voy a anotarlo en su gráfica y a informar a la enfermera de inmediato.
¿Debemos suspender la pastilla por ahora?
No, por favor siga dándosela, pero la enfermera lo llamará hoy para evaluarlo.

English translation:
I've noticed he's been more drowsy since he started the new medication.
Yes, I will note it in his chart and inform the nurse immediately.
Should we stop the pill for now?
No, please continue giving it to him, but the nurse will call you today to evaluate it.

Practice Scenario

La auxiliar Rosa notó que el señor López tenía más confusión y una nueva erupción cutánea. Inmediatamente documentó los cambios en su hoja de reporte y se lo informó a la enfermera supervisora. Describió con detalle los síntomas observados para una evaluación rápida, asegurándose de que el residente recibiera la atención médica necesaria con prontitud y respeto.

English translation:
The aide Rosa noticed Mr. Lopez had increased confusion and a new skin rash. She immediately documented the changes on his report sheet and informed the supervising nurse. She described the observed symptoms in detail for a quick evaluation, ensuring the resident received the necessary medical attention

promptly and respectfully.

MANAGING
MEDICATION REFILLS

¿Necesita un refill de su medicina? - neh-seh-SEE-tah oon reh-FEEL deh soo meh-dee-SEE-nah - Do you need a refill of your medicine?

La receta - lah reh-SEH-tah - The prescription

¿Podemos llamar a su farmacia? - poh-DEH-mohs yah-MAHR ah soo fahr-MAH-see-ah - Can we call your pharmacy?

Suplemento - soo-pleh-MEN-toh - Supplement

¿Toma esta pastilla con comida? - TOH-mah EH-stah pahs-TEE-yah kohn koh-MEE-dah - Do you take this pill with food?

¿Tiene suficiente medicina? - tee-EH-neh soo-fee-SYEN-teh meh-dee-SEE-nah - Do you have enough medicine?

¿Le duele algo? - leh doo-EH-leh AHL-goh - Are you in any pain?

¿A qué hora toma su medicina? - ah keh OH-rah TOH-mah soo meh-dee-SEE-nah - What time do you take your medicine?

¿Puedo ayudarle con sus pastillas? - PWEH-doh ah-yoo-DAHR-leh kohn soos pahs-TEE-yahs - Can I help you with your pills?

¿Necesita ayuda para ordenar sus medicamentos? - neh-seh-SEE-tah ah-YOO-dah PAH-rah ohr-deh-NAHR soos meh-dee-kah-MEN-tohs - Do you need help organizing your medications?

¿Tuvo efectos secundarios? - TOO-boh eh-FEK-tohs seh-koon-DAH-ree-ohs - Did you have any side effects?

Don/Doña - dohn / DOH-nyah - Mr./Mrs. (a respectful title)

Grammatical Examples

Necesito el frasco de pastillas. - I need the bottle of pills.

Busco la caja de pastillas. - I am looking for the box of pills.

Reviso la bolsa de pastillas. - I check the bag of pills.

Lleno la receta para el señor. - I fill the prescription for the gentleman.

Lleno la receta para la señora. - I fill the prescription for the lady.

Confirmo la dosis con la enfermera. - I confirm the dose with the nurse.

Confirmo la dosis con el enfermero. - I confirm the dose with the nurse.

Anoto la hora en la hoja. - I write down the time on the sheet.

Practice Dialog

Buenos días, veo que las pastillas para la presión de la señora se están acabando. ¿Quiere que llame a la farmacia para solicitar el refill?

Sí, por favor. ¿Podría también confirmar con el doctor la receta? No estoy segura de si necesita una nueva autorización.

Claro que sí. Les llamo ahora mismo y le aviso cuando esté listo para recoger.

Muchas gracias. Usted siempre está muy atenta a estos detalles.

English translation:

Good morning, I see that the lady's blood pressure pills are running out. Would you like me to call the pharmacy to request the refill?

Yes, please. Could you also confirm the prescription with the doctor? I'm not sure if it needs a new authorization.

Of course. I'll call them right now and let you know when it's ready for pickup.

Thank you very much. You are always very attentive to these details.

Practice Scenario

La enfermera revisa las recetas mensuales. Doña Carmen necesita un nuevo frasco de pastillas para la presión. La auxiliar confirma la autorización con el médico. Luego, llama a la farmacia para solicitar el reabastecimiento. Cuando llega, verifica la medicación contra la hoja de administración. Le entrega el frasco a la enfermera con una sonrisa, asegurando el cuidado continuo de la residente.

English translation: The nurse reviews the monthly prescriptions. Doña Carmen needs a new bottle of blood pressure pills. The aide confirms the authorization with the doctor. Then, she calls the pharmacy to request the refill. When it arrives, she verifies the medication against the administration sheet. She hands the bottle to the nurse with a smile, ensuring the resident's continuous care.

DISCUSSING PAIN MANAGEMENT OPTIONS

¿Dónde le duele? - DOHN-deh leh DWEL-eh - Where does it hurt?

¿Puede describir el dolor? - PWEH-deh deh-SKREE-beer ehl doh-LOHR - Can you describe the pain?

Voy a traer su medicina - Voy ah trah-EHR soo meh-dee-SEE-nah - I am going to get your medicine

¿Le gustaría un calmante? - Leh goos-tah-REE-ah oon kahl-MAHN-teh - Would you like a pain reliever?

Vamos a intentar una posición más cómoda - VAH-mohs ah een-ten-TAHR OO-nah poh-see-SYOHN mahs KOH-moh-dah - Let's try a more comfortable position

Señora/Señor, ¿así está mejor? - seh-NYOH-rah / seh-NYOHR, ah-SEE ehs-TAH meh-HOR - Ma'am/Sir, is this better?

Es hora de su medicamento para el dolor - Ehs OH-rah deh soo meh-dee-kah-MEN-toh PAH-rah ehl doh-LOHR - It's time for your pain medication

¿Le ayuda la almohada? - Leh ah-YOO-dah lah ahl-moh-AH-dah - Does the pillow help you?

Voy a aplicar hielo para la hinchazón - Voy ah ah-plee-KAHR YEH-loh PAH-rah lah een-chah-SOHN - I am going to apply ice for the swelling

¿Le alivia el masaje? - Leh ah-LEE-vyah ehl mah-SAH-heh - Does the massage relieve it for you?

Vamos a moverle con cuidado - VAH-mohs ah moh-BEHR-leh kohn kwee-DAH-doh - We are going to move you carefully

¿Necesita algo más para estar cómodo/a? - Neh-seh-SEE-tah AHL-goh mahs PAH-rah ehs-TAHR KOH-moh-doh/dah - Do you need anything else to be comfortable?

Grammatical Examples

¿Le duele la espalda? - Does your back hurt?

¿Le duelen las rodillas? - Do your knees hurt?

¿Le duele el hombro? - Does your shoulder hurt?

¿Le duelen las articulaciones? - Do your joints hurt?

Practice Dialog

Veo que está incómodo. ¿Le gustaría que probemos con el medicamento para el dolor ahora o prefiere primero intentar con una compresa tibia?

Creo que primero probemos con la compresa. A veces el calor me ayuda bastante.

Perfecto. Voy a prepararla ahora mismo. Si en media hora no se siente mejor, podemos hablar de la medicina.

Gracias. Le aviso si no hay cambio.

English translation:

I see you're uncomfortable. Would you like to try the pain medication now, or would you prefer to try a warm compress first?

I think we try the compress first. The heat sometimes helps me a lot.

Perfect. I'll prepare it right now. If in half an hour you don't feel better, we can talk about the medicine.

Thank you. I'll let you know if there's no change.

Practice Scenario

La Sra. García se quejaba de dolor en su artritis. Yo, su auxiliar de enfermería, revisé su historial de medicamentos. Le ofrecí su analgésico recetado según el horario, pero también sugerí una bolsa de agua caliente para sus articulaciones. Ella aceptó ambas opciones. Documenté su queja y la respuesta en su informe para el equipo de cuidado.

English translation:

Mrs. Garcia complained of arthritis pain. I, her nursing assistant, checked her medication record. I offered her prescribed painkiller on schedule, but also suggested a hot water bottle for her joints. She accepted both options. I documented her complaint and the response in her report for the care team.

MEAL PLANNING AND DIETARY RESTRICTIONS

¿Qué le gustaría comer? - keh leh goos-tah-REE-ah koh-MEHR - What would you like to eat?

¿Tiene alguna alergia? - TYEH-neh ahl-GOO-nah ah-LEHR-hyah - Do you have any allergies?

¿Puede masticar esto? - PWEH-deh mahs-tee-KAHR EHS-toh - Can you chew this?

Necesita una dieta blanda - neh-seh-SEE-tah OO-nah DYEH-tah BLAHN-dah - You need a soft diet

Sin sal - seen sahl - Without salt

Bajo en azúcar - BAH-hoh ehn ah-SOO-kahr - Low in sugar

Vamos a tomar los líquidos - VAH-mohs ah toh-MAHR lohs LEE-kee-dohs - Let's drink the liquids

¿Tiene sed? - TYEH-neh sed - Are you thirsty?

Vamos a comer despacio - VAH-mohs ah koh-MEHR des-PAH-syoh - Let's eat slowly

¿Le duele el estómago? - Leh DWEH-leh el ehs-TOH-mah-goh - Does your stomach hurt?

¿Le gusta el té? - Leh GOOS-tah el teh - Do you like tea?

Es hora de la merienda - ehs OH-rah deh lah meh-RYEN-dah - It is time for a snack

La señora García necesita una dieta baja en sodio. - Mrs. Garcia

71

needs a low-sodium diet.

El señor Martínez necesita una dieta blanda. - Mr. Martinez needs a soft diet.

La residente necesita una comida sin gluten. - The resident needs a gluten-free meal.

El paciente necesita líquidos claros esta tarde. - The patient needs clear liquids this afternoon.

La señora López necesita ayuda para cortar la carne. - Mrs. Lopez needs help cutting the meat.

Practice Dialog

Para planear las comidas de esta semana, ¿hay algún alimento que no pueda comer o que le cause molestias?

Sí, por favor eviten las comidas muy saladas. El médico dijo que debo cuidar la presión arterial.

Perfecto, anotado. Prepararemos todo bajo en sodio. ¿Le gustan las sopas de verduras?

Sí, me encantan. Muchas gracias por preguntar.

English translation:

To plan the meals for this week, is there any food you cannot eat or that causes you discomfort?

Yes, please avoid very salty foods. The doctor said I must watch my blood pressure.

Perfect, noted. We will prepare everything low in sodium. Do you like vegetable soups?

Yes, I love them. Thank you very much for asking.

Practice Scenario

La señora García rechazó la cena. La CNA, recordando su nueva dieta para disfagia, le ofreció el puré de pollo con verduras espesado. Con paciencia, la animó: "Pruebe un poco, es su favorito". La señora comió lentamente. La CNA documentó la ingesta en el gráfico de alimentación, satisfecha por asegurar su nutrición dentro de las restricciones prescritas.

English translation: Mrs. Garcia refused dinner. The CNA,

recalling her new diet for dysphagia, offered her the thickened pureed chicken with vegetables. Patiently, she encouraged her: "Try a bit, it's your favorite." The woman ate slowly. The CNA documented the intake on the flow sheet, satisfied to ensure her nutrition within the prescribed restrictions.

ASSISTING WITH EATING AND DRINKING

¿Le gustaría comer? - leh goos-tah-REE-ah koh-MEHR - Would you like to eat?

¿Le gustaría beber? - leh goos-tah-REE-ah beh-BEHR - Would you like to drink?

Vamos a tomar un poco de agua - VAH-mohs ah toh-MAR oon POH-koh deh AH-gwah - Let's drink a little water

¿Necesita ayuda? - neh-seh-SEE-tah ah-YOO-dah - Do you need help?

Abra la boca, por favor - AH-brah lah BOH-kah pohr fah-VOHR - Open your mouth, please

Mastique despacio - mahs-TEE-keh dehs-PAH-syoh - Chew slowly

Trague con cuidado - TRAH-geh kohn kwee-DAH-doh - Swallow carefully

Tenga cuidado, está caliente - TEN-gah kwee-DAH-doh ehs-TAH kah-lee-EN-teh - Be careful, it's hot

¿Está cómodo/a? - ehs-TAH KOH-moh-doh/dah - Are you comfortable?

¿Tiene hambre? - tee-EN-eh AHM-breh - Are you hungry?

¿Tiene sed? - tee-EN-eh SEHD - Are you thirsty?

Buen provecho - bwehn proh-VEH-choh - Enjoy your meal

Grammatical Examples

¿Le gustaría más agua? - Would you like more water?
¿Le gustaría más jugo? - Would you like more juice?
¿Le gustaría más té? - Would you like more tea?
¿Le gustaría más sopa? - Would you like more soup?

Practice Dialog

Ya llegó su almuerzo, señora. ¿Le ayudo a sentarse un poco más?
Sí, por favor. Tengo un poco de sed.
Primero le doy un poco de agua. Aquí tiene, tome pequeños sorbos.
Gracias. Eso está mucho mejor.

Practice Scenario

La señora Rosa acepta la cuchara lentamente. Su apetito es variable. Le ofrezco pequeños sips de agua entre bocados para evitar la deshidratación. Hablo con calma, recordándole los sabores. A veces gira la cabeza, y respeto su decisión de parar. Mi prioridad es su seguridad y dignidad durante la asistencia con la alimentación.

English translation: Mrs. Rosa accepts the spoon slowly. Her appetite is variable. I offer her small sips of water between bites to prevent dehydration. I speak calmly, reminding her of the flavors. Sometimes she turns her head, and I respect her decision to stop. My priority is her safety and dignity during mealtime assistance.

MANAGING DIABETES AND SPECIAL DIETS

¿Necesita ayuda para medir su azúcar? - NEH-seh-see-tah ah-YOO-dah pah-rah meh-DEER soo ah-SOO-kahr - Do you need help checking your sugar?

Vamos a revisar su azúcar en la sangre - VAH-mohs ah reh-bee-SAHR soo ah-SOO-kahr ehn lah SAHN-greh - Let's check your blood sugar

Es hora de su medicina para la diabetes - ehs OH-rah deh soo meh-dee-SEE-nah pah-rah lah dee-ah-BEH-tehs - It's time for your diabetes medicine

¿Tiene sed o hambre? - tee-EH-neh SEHD oh AHM-breh - Are you thirsty or hungry?

Vamos a comer algo saludable - VAH-mohs ah koh-MEHR AHL-goh sah-loo-DAH-bleh - Let's eat something healthy

¿Le duele algún dedo del pie? - leh doo-EH-leh ahl-GOON DEH-doh dehl pee-EH - Does any toe hurt?

Por favor, mantenga la dieta - pohr fah-VOHR, mahn-TEHN-gah lah dee-EH-tah - Please, maintain the diet

Necesita beber más agua - neh-seh-SEE-tah beh-BEHR mahs AH-gwah - You need to drink more water

¿Le gustaría una merienda baja en azúcar? - leh goos-tah-REE-ah OO-nah meh-ree-EN-dah BAH-hah ehn ah-SOO-kahr - Would you like a low-sugar snack?

Vamos a cuidar sus pies - VAH-mohs ah kwee-DAHR soos pee-EHS - Let's take care of your feet

¿Se siente mareado o débil? - seh see-EN-teh mah-reh-AH-doh oh

DEH-beel - Do you feel dizzy or weak?

Es importante no saltarse las comidas - ehs eem-pohr-TAHN-teh noh sahl-TAHR-seh lahs koh-MEE-dahs - It is important not to skip meals

Grammatical Examples

El residente necesita su medicamento para la diabetes. - The resident needs his diabetes medication.

La residente necesita su medicamento para la diabetes. - The resident needs her diabetes medication.

El señor Martínez necesita su medicamento para la diabetes. - Mr. Martinez needs his diabetes medication.

La señora García necesita su medicamento para la diabetes. - Mrs. Garcia needs her diabetes medication.

El paciente necesita su medicamento para la diabetes. - The patient needs his diabetes medication.

La paciente necesita su medicamento para la diabetes. - The patient needs her diabetes medication.

Practice Dialog

Ya tomé su azúcar, está en 95. ¿Le gustaría su merienda de la tarde ahora?

Perfecto, sí. ¿Podría traerme el yogur sin azúcar y las galletas integrales, por favor?

Claro que sí. Aquí tiene. También le traje un vaso de agua para que se mantenga hidratado.

Muchas gracias por recordármelo. Es importante seguir el plan para sentirme bien.

English translation:

I already took your sugar, it's at 95. Would you like your afternoon snack now?

Perfect, yes. Could you bring me the sugar-free yogurt and the whole-wheat crackers, please?

Of course. Here you go. I also brought you a glass of water to keep you hydrated.

Thank you so much for reminding me. It's important to follow the plan to feel well.

La señora García, con diabetes, a veces se niega a comer su dieta especial. La auxiliar de enfermería, Elena, le explica con paciencia la importancia de cada alimento en su bandeja. Le ofrece el puré de manzana sin azúcar que le gusta. Monitorea su glucemia con respeto, asegurándose de que doña García se sienta cuidada y comprendida en su rutina de cuidados.

English translation:
Mrs. Garcia, who has diabetes, sometimes refuses to eat her special diet. The nursing assistant, Elena, patiently explains the importance of each food on her tray. She offers her the sugar-free applesauce that she likes. She monitors her blood glucose with respect, ensuring Mrs. Garcia feels cared for and understood in her care routine.

ENCOURAGING HYDRATION

¿Le gustaría un poco de agua? - leh goos-tah-REE-ah oon POH-koh deh AH-gwah - Would you like some water?

Es importante mantenerse hidratado/a - ehs eem-por-TAHN-teh mahn-teh-NEHR-seh ee-drah-TAH-doh/dah - It is important to stay hydrated

Vamos a tomar un sorbo - VAH-mohs ah toh-MAHR oon SOHR-boh - Let's take a sip

¿Puedo llenar su vaso? - PWEH-doh yeh-NAHR soo VAH-soh - May I fill your glass?

Para sentirse mejor - PAH-rah sen-TEER-seh meh-HOR - To feel better

Tenga esto, por favor - TEN-gah EHS-toh por fah-VOR - Have this, please

Le ayudará a sentirse bien - leh ah-yoo-dah-RAH ah sen-TEER-seh bee-EN - It will help you feel well

Un poco más - oon POH-koh mahs - A little bit more

Muy bien, así - MOO-ee bee-EN, ah-SEE - Very good, like that

¿Tiene sed? - tee-EH-neh sed - Are you thirsty?

Mantengamos sus líquidos altos - mahn-ten-GAH-mohs soos LEE-kee-dohs AHL-tohs - Let's keep your fluids up

¿Prefiere agua o jugo? - preh-fee-EH-reh AH-gwah oh HOO-goh - Do you prefer water or juice?

Grammatical Examples

¿Le gustaría un vaso de agua? - Would you like a glass of water?

¿Le gustaría una taza de té? - Would you like a cup of tea?
¿Le gustaría un poco de jugo? - Would you like some juice?
¿Le gustaría un sorbo de esto? - Would you like a sip of this?

Practice Dialog

Ya veo que su botella de agua está casi llena. ¿Le gustaría tomar unos sorbos antes de que continuemos?

Tiene razón, siempre se me olvida. Pero no tengo mucha sed.

Entiendo, es común. Beber un poco ahora nos ayudará a evitar que se sienta mareado más tarde.

Tiene sentido. Mejor prevenir que lamentar, ¿verdad? Le haré caso.

English translation:

I see your water bottle is still quite full. Would you like to take a few sips before we continue?

You're right, I always forget. But I'm not very thirsty.

I understand, that's common. Drinking a little now will help us avoid you feeling dizzy later.

That makes sense. Better safe than sorry, right? I'll listen to you.

Practice Scenario

La señora Rosa rechazó el vaso de agua. María, su auxiliar de enfermería, recordó su consejo. En lugar de insistir, ofreció una taza de su té favorito con una pajita. "Para mantenernos hidratadas, señora", dijo con una sonrisa. Rosa bebió lentamente. María anotó la ingesta en el registro, satisfecha con esta pequeña victoria para la salud de su paciente.

English translation: Mrs. Rosa refused the glass of water. María, her nursing assistant, remembered her advice. Instead of insisting, she offered a cup of her favorite tea with a straw. "To keep us hydrated, ma'am," she said with a smile. Rosa drank slowly. María noted the intake on the chart, satisfied with this small victory for her patient's health.

DISCUSSING APPETITE CHANGES

Key Vocabulary

¿Le apetece algo de comer? - leh ah-peh-TEH-seh AHL-goh deh koh-MEHR - Would you like something to eat?

¿Tiene hambre? - TYEH-neh AHM-breh - Are you hungry?

¿Tiene sed? - TYEH-neh SEHD - Are you thirsty?

¿Le gustaría probar esto? - leh goos-tah-REE-ah proh-BAHR EHS-toh - Would you like to try this?

¿Prefiere algo diferente? - preh-fyeh-reh AHL-goh dee-feh-REHN-teh - Would you prefer something different?

Su apetito - soo ah-peh-TEE-toh - Your appetite

¿Le sabe bien la comida? - leh SAH-beh byehn lah koh-MEE-dah - Does the food taste good to you?

¿Le duele algo al comer? - leh DWEH-leh AHL-goh ahl koh-MEHR - Does anything hurt when you eat?

¿Le cuesta tragar? - leh KWEHS-tah trah-GAHR - Is it difficult for you to swallow?

Bocadito - boh-kah-DEE-toh - Small bite

Para mantenerse fuerte - PAH-rah mahn-teh-NEHR-seh FWEHR-teh - To keep your strength up

Por favor, tome un poco más - pohr fah-BOHR, TOH-meh oon POH-koh mahs - Please, have a little more

Grammatical Examples

¿Ha comido bien hoy, señor García? - Have you eaten well today, Mr. Garcia?

¿Ha comido bien hoy, señora López? - Have you eaten well today,

Mrs. Lopez?

¿Ha comido bien hoy, señorita Ruiz? - Have you eaten well today, Miss Ruiz?

Practice Dialog

He notado que ha estado comiendo menos de lo habitual últimamente.

Sí, la verdad es que no tengo mucho apetito desde que empecé con la nueva medicina.

Entiendo. ¿Le parece si probamos con porciones más pequeñas, pero más seguidas durante el día?

Eso suena bien. Así no me siento abrumada con el plato lleno.

English translation:

I've noticed you've been eating less than usual lately.

Yes, the truth is I haven't had much of an appetite since I started the new medicine.

I understand. What if we try smaller portions, but more frequently throughout the day?

That sounds good. That way I don't feel overwhelmed with a full plate.

Practice Scenario

La señora García rechazó el desayuno otra vez. "No tengo hambre", murmuró. En lugar de insistir, le ofrecí un batido nutricional y le pregunté sobre su rutina de medicación. Noté que estaba estreñida. Reporté los cambios de apetito y estreñimiento a la enfermera para ajustar su plan de cuidado, asegurándome de que reciba la nutrición que necesita.

English translation:

Mrs. Garcia refused breakfast again. "I'm not hungry," she murmured. Instead of insisting, I offered her a nutritional shake and asked about her medication routine. I noted she was constipated. I reported the appetite changes and constipation to the nurse to adjust her care plan, ensuring she gets the nutrition she needs.

TAKING VITAL SIGNS (TEMPERATURE, BLOOD PRESSURE)

¿Cómo se siente hoy? - KOH-moh seh SYEN-teh oy - How are you feeling today?

Voy a tomarle la temperatura - voy ah toh-mar-leh lah tem-peh-rah-TOO-rah - I am going to take your temperature

¿Puede levantar la manga, por favor? - PWEH-deh leh-van-TAR lah MAN-gah por fah-VOR - Can you lift your sleeve, please?

Voy a tomarle la presión - voy ah toh-mar-leh lah preh-SYON - I am going to take your blood pressure

Respire profundamente - res-PEE-reh pro-fun-dah-MEN-teh - Breathe deeply

Quieto, por favor - KYEH-toh por fah-VOR - Hold still, please

Abra la boca - AH-brah lah BOH-kah - Open your mouth

¿Tiene dolor? - TYEH-neh doh-LOR - Are you in pain?

Necesito escuchar su corazón - neh-seh-SEE-toh es-koo-CHAR soo ko-rah-SON - I need to listen to your heart

¿Puede sentarse aquí? - PWEH-deh sen-TAR-seh ah-KEE - Can you sit here, please?

Gracias por su cooperación - GRAH-syahs por soo koh-op-eh-rah-SYON - Thank you for your cooperation

¿Necesita algo más? - neh-seh-SEE-tah AHL-goh mas - Do you need anything else?

Grammatical Examples

Voy a tomarle la temperatura. - I am going to take your temperature.

Voy a tomarle la presión arterial. - I am going to take your blood pressure.

Voy a ayudarle a sentarse. - I am going to help you sit up.

Voy a revisarle el brazo. - I am going to check your arm.

Voy a explicarle el procedimiento. - I am going to explain the procedure to you.

Practice Dialog

Buenos días, voy a tomarle la temperatura y la presión arterial, ¿le parece bien?

Sí, claro. ¿Necesito hacer algo en especial?

No, solo relájese y apoye el brazo, por favor. Empezaré con la temperatura.

Perfecto, avíseme si necesita que me mueva de alguna manera.

English translation:

Good morning, I'm going to take your temperature and blood pressure, is that alright?

Yes, of course. Do I need to do anything special?

No, just relax and rest your arm, please. I'll start with the temperature.

Perfect, let me know if you need me to move in any way.

Practice Scenario

La enfermera auxiliar mide los signos vitales de la señora Elena. Toma su temperatura con el termómetro timpánico y su presión arterial con el baumanómetro. Mientras, conversa amablemente con ella para mantenerla tranquila. Registra los valores en la gráfica, notando una leve febrícula. Le ofrece agua y le asegura que volverá pronto para monitorearla.

English translation:

The nursing assistant measures Mrs. Elena's vital signs. She takes her temperature with the tympanic thermometer and her blood pressure with the sphygmomanometer. Meanwhile, she chats kindly with her to keep her calm. She records the values on the chart, noting a slight fever. She offers her water and assures her she will return soon to monitor her.

MONITORING BLOOD SUGAR LEVELS

Key Vocabulary

¿Cómo se siente hoy? - KOH-moh seh see-EN-teh oy - How do you feel today?

Vamos a revisar su azúcar - VAH-mohs ah reh-vee-SAHR soo ah-SOO-kahr - We are going to check your sugar

Necesito una gota de sangre - neh-seh-SEE-toh OO-nah GOH-tah deh SAHN-greh - I need a drop of blood

Por favor, limpie su dedo - por fah-VOR, LEEM-pee-eh soo DEH-doh - Please, clean your finger

Va a sentir un pequeño pinchazo - vah ah sen-TEER oon peh-KEH-nyoh peen-CHAH-soh - You will feel a small poke

Mantenga su mano quieta - mahn-TEN-gah soo MAH-noh kee-EH-tah - Keep your hand still

¿Cuándo comió por última vez? - KWAHN-doh koh-mee-OH por OOL-tee-mah ves - When did you last eat?

¿Tuvo su medicina para la diabetes? - TOO-voh soo meh-dee-SEE-nah PAH-rah lah dee-ah-BEH-tes - Did you have your diabetes medicine?

Su nivel de azúcar es... - soo nee-VEL deh ah-SOO-kahr es - Your sugar level is...

Está un poco alto/bajo - es-TAH oon POH-koh AHL-toh/BAH-hoh - It is a little high/low

¿Tiene hambre o sed? - tee-EH-neh AHM-breh oh sed - Are you hungry or thirsty?

Voy a anotar el resultado - voy ah ah-noh-TAR el reh-sool-TAH-doh - I am going to write down the result

Grammatical Examples

Necesito revisar su nivel de azúcar. - I need to check your blood sugar level.

Él necesita revisar su nivel de azúcar. - He needs to check his blood sugar level.

Ella necesita revisar su nivel de azúcar. - She needs to check her blood sugar level.

Usted necesita revisar su nivel de azúcar. - You (formal) need to check your blood sugar level.

Nosotros necesitamos revisar su nivel de azúcar. - We need to check your blood sugar level.

Ellos necesitan revisar su nivel de azúcar. - They need to check their blood sugar level.

Practice Dialog

Buenos días, es hora de revisar el nivel de azúcar en la sangre.
Por supuesto, la lanceta es nueva y apenas sentirá un pinchacito.
Gracias por avisarme. ¿Los números están bien?
Sí, están en un rango perfecto. Ahora puede tomar su desayuno.

English translation:
Good morning, it's time to check your blood sugar level.
Of course, the lancet is new and you will barely feel a prick.
Thank you for warning me. Are the numbers okay?
Yes, they are in a perfect range. Now you can have your breakfast.

Practice Scenario

La enfermera auxiliar revisa la glucosa de la señora Elena después del desayuno. El nivel está alto. Con paciencia, la auxiliar le pregunta sobre su comida y le recuerda la importancia de la dieta. Juntas revisan el menú para el almuerzo, eligiendo opciones más balanceadas. La señora Elena asiente, agradecida por el cuidado respetuoso en su hogar de ancianos.

English translation:

The nursing assistant checks Mrs. Elena's glucose after breakfast. The level is high. patiently, the aide asks her about her meal and reminds her of the importance of diet. Together they review the menu for lunch, choosing more balanced options. Mrs. Elena nods, grateful for the respectful care in her nursing home.

OBSERVING AND REPORTING HEALTH CHANGES

Key Vocabulary

¿Cómo se siente hoy? - KOH-moh seh see-EN-teh oy - How do you feel today?

¿Tiene dolor? - tee-EH-neh doh-LOHR - Do you have pain?

¿Dónde le duele? - DOHN-deh leh doo-EH-leh - Where does it hurt?

Necesita usar el baño - neh-seh-SEE-tah oo-SAHR el BAH-nyoh - You need to use the bathroom

Vamos a tomar sus signos vitales - VAH-mohs ah toh-MAHR soos SEEG-nohs vee-TAH-lehs - Let's take your vital signs

Su temperatura - soo tem-peh-rah-TOO-rah - Your temperature

Presión arterial - preh-see-ON ahr-teh-ree-AHL - Blood pressure

¿Le duele aquí? - leh doo-EH-leh ah-KEE - Does it hurt here?

¿Tiene dificultad para respirar? - tee-EH-neh dee-fee-kool-TAHD PAH-rah res-pee-RAHR - Do you have difficulty breathing?

Está mareado/a - eh-STAH mah-reh-AH-doh/dah - You are dizzy

¿Cómo durmió anoche? - KOH-moh door-MEE-oh ah-NOH-cheh - How did you sleep last night?

Voy a reportar esto a la enfermera - voy ah reh-por-TAHR EHS-toh ah lah en-fer-MEH-rah - I am going to report this to the nurse

Grammatical Examples

El señor parece confundido hoy. - The gentleman seems confused today.

La señora parece confundida hoy. - The lady seems confused today.

El residente parece cansado esta mañana. - The resident (male) seems tired this morning.

La residente parece cansada esta mañana. - The resident (female) seems tired this morning.

El paciente parece débil. - The patient (male) seems weak.

La paciente parece débil. - The patient (female) seems weak.

Practice Dialog

Buenos días, noté que está tosiendo más hoy y parece que le cuesta respirar.

Sí, desde anoche siento el pecho más cargado y me canso al hablar.

Voy a tomarle la temperatura y la saturación de oxígeno, y luego llamaremos a la enfermera.

Gracias, se lo agradezco. Me tiene un poco preocupado.

English translation:
Good morning, I noticed you're coughing more today and seem to be having trouble breathing.

Yes, since last night my chest feels more congested and I get tired when I talk.

I'm going to take your temperature and oxygen saturation, and then we'll call the nurse.

Thank you, I appreciate it. I'm a little worried.

Practice Scenario

La auxiliar nota que el señor López, normalmente conversador, está inusualmente somnoliento y con la piel caliente. Inmediatamente mide sus signos vitales: fiebre y taquicardia. Documenta meticulosamente los cambios en su estado y reporta sus observaciones a la enfermera. Su supervisora valora su vigilancia, crucial para una intervención temprana en el adulto mayor.

English translation:

The aide notices that Mr. Lopez, normally talkative, is unusually drowsy and has warm skin. She immediately takes his vital signs: fever and tachycardia. She meticulously documents the changes in his condition and reports her observations to the nurse. Her supervisor values her vigilance, crucial for early intervention in the elderly.

WOUND CARE AND DRESSING CHANGES

Voy a limpiar su herida - voy ah leem-PEE-ahr soo eh-REE-dah - I am going to clean your wound

Necesito cambiar el vendaje - neh-seh-SEE-toh kahm-bee-AHR el ven-DAH-heh - I need to change the dressing

Voy a ser muy cuidadoso/a - voy ah sehr MOO-ee kwee-dah-DOH-soh/sah - I am going to be very careful

¿Le duele aquí? - leh doo-EH-leh ah-KEE - Does it hurt here?

Por favor, quédese quieto/a - por fah-VOR, KEH-deh-seh kee-EH-toh/tah - Please, keep still

Esto va a ayudar a prevenir una infección - EHS-toh vah ah ah-yoo-DAHR ah preh-veh-NEER OO-nah een-fek-see-ON - This will help prevent an infection

La herida se ve mejor - lah eh-REE-dah seh veh meh-HOR - The wound looks better

Vamos a levantarle suavemente - VAH-mohs ah leh-vahn-TAHR-leh swah-veh-MEN-teh - We are going to lift you gently

¿Puede mover esto para mí? - PWEH-deh moh-VEHR EHS-toh PAH-rah MEE - Can you move this for me?

Señor/Señora - sen-YOR / sen-YOR-ah - Sir/Ma'am

Gracias por su paciencia - GRAH-see-ahs por soo pah-see-EN-see-ah - Thank you for your patience

Está sanando muy bien - ehs-TAH sah-NAN-doh MOO-ee bee-EN - It is healing very well

La herida está limpia. - The wound is clean.
La venda está limpia. - The bandage is clean.
La piel está limpia. - The skin is clean.
La gasa está limpia. - The gauze is clean.
El apósito está limpio. - The dressing is clean.
El vendaje está limpio. - The bandage is clean.
El área está limpia. - The area is clean.

Practice Dialog

Voy a limpiar su herida con una solución salina para prevenir una infección.

¿Le duele o siente alguna molestia?

No, no duele. ¿Es normal que tenga un poco de secreción?

Sí, es normal. Es parte del proceso de curación. Avíseme inmediatamente si ve enrojecimiento o si la secreción aumenta.

English translation:

I am going to clean your wound with a saline solution to prevent an infection.

Does it hurt or do you feel any discomfort?

No, it doesn't hurt. Is it normal to have a little bit of drainage?

Yes, it's normal. It's part of the healing process. Tell me immediately if you see redness or if the drainage increases.

Practice Scenario

La enfermera examina la úlcera por presión en el talón del residente. Limpia la herida con solución salina suavemente, aplica una pomada antibiótica y coloca un apósito nuevo de espuma. Le explica al señor López cada paso para mantenerlo tranquilo. Le recuerda la importancia de cambiar de posición frecuentemente para ayudar en la cicatrización.

English translation: The nurse examines the pressure ulcer on the resident's heel. She cleans the wound with saline gently, applies antibiotic ointment, and places a new foam dressing. She explains each step to Mr. Lopez to keep him calm. She reminds him of the importance of changing position frequently to aid healing.

RECOGNIZING SIGNS OF ILLNESS OR DISTRESS

Key Vocabulary

¿Cómo se siente hoy? - KOH-moh seh SYEN-teh oy - How do you feel today?

¿Tiene dolor? - TYEH-neh doh-LOHR - Do you have pain?

¿Dónde le duele? - DOHN-deh leh DWEH-leh - Where does it hurt?

¿Necesita ir al baño? - neh-seh-SEE-tah eer ahl BAH-nyoh - Do you need to go to the bathroom?

¿Le duele la cabeza? - leh DWEH-leh lah kah-BEH-sah - Does your head hurt?

¿Tiene fiebre? - TYEH-neh FYEH-breh - Do you have a fever?

¿Se siente mareado/a? - seh SYEN-teh mah-reh-AH-doh/dah - Do you feel dizzy?

¿Tiene dificultad para respirar? - TYEH-neh dee-fee-kool-TAHD pah-rah res-pee-RAHR - Do you have difficulty breathing?

Vamos a tomar su temperatura - VAH-mohs ah toh-MAHR soo tem-peh-rah-TOO-rah - Let's take your temperature

¿Puede mostrarme dónde le duele? - PWEH-deh mohs-TRAHR-meh DOHN-deh leh DWEH-leh - Can you show me where it hurts?

¿Necesita su medicina? - neh-seh-SEE-tah soo meh-dee-SEE-nah - Do you need your medicine?

Señor/Señora - seh-NYOHR/seh-NYOH-rah - Sir/Ma'am

Grammatical Examples

El señor parece confundido. - The gentleman seems confused.

La señora parece confundida. - The lady seems confused.

El residente parece inquieto. - The resident (male) seems restless.

La residente parece inquieta. - The resident (female) seems restless.

El paciente parece débil. - The patient (male) seems weak.

La paciente parece débil. - The patient (female) seems weak.

Practice Dialog

¿Señora, cómo se siente hoy? Noté que no terminó su desayuno.

No tengo mucho apetito y me duele un poco la cabeza.

Voy a tomarle la temperatura. También, ¿le gustaría que llamemos a su hija?

Sí, por favor. Y ¿podría traerme un vaso de agua? Me siento un poco débil.

English translation:

Ma'am, how are you feeling today? I noticed you didn't finish your breakfast.

I don't have much of an appetite and I have a bit of a headache.

I'm going to take your temperature. Also, would you like us to call your daughter?

Yes, please. And could you bring me a glass of water? I feel a little weak.

Practice Scenario

La señora García, normalmente conversadora, estaba callada y rechazaba el desayuno. La auxiliar de enfermería notó su piel pálida y le preguntó con calma sobre su malestar. Al tomar sus signos vitales, detectó fiebre. Reportó sus observaciones a la enfermera de inmediato, asegurándose de que la residente recibiera una pronta evaluación médica por el posible cambio en su condición.

English translation: Mrs. Garcia, normally talkative, was quiet and refused breakfast. The nursing assistant noticed her pale skin and calmly asked about her discomfort. Upon taking her vital signs, she detected a fever. She reported her observations to the nurse immediately, ensuring the resident received a prompt medical evaluation for the potential change in her condition.

PROVIDING COMFORT DURING ANXIETY OR CONFUSION

Está bien - ehs-TAH byehn - It's okay

Respire profundamente - rehs-PEE-reh proh-foon-dah-MEN-teh - Breathe deeply

Estoy aquí para ayudarle - ehs-TOY ah-KEE pah-rah ah-yoo-DAHR-leh - I am here to help you

Tómese su tiempo - TOH-meh-seh soo TYEHM-poh - Take your time

Voy a quedarme con usted - BOY ah keh-DAHR-meh kohn oos-TEHD - I am going to stay with you

¿Necesita algo? - neh-seh-SEE-tah AHL-goh - Do you need anything?

Está a salvo - ehs-TAH ah SAHL-boh - You are safe

Descanse - dehs-KAHN-seh - Rest

Todo está bien - TOH-doh ehs-TAH byehn - Everything is okay

Le entiendo - leh en-TYEN-doh - I understand you

¿Le gustaría un poco de agua? - leh goos-tah-REE-ah oon POH-koh deh AH-gwah - Would you like some water?

Tranquilo/Tranquila (use based on patient's gender) - trahn-KEE-loh / trahn-KEE-lah - Calm (masculine/feminine)

Grammatical Examples

Usted está a salvo aquí. - You are safe here.

Usted está en su hogar. - You are at your home.

Usted está con personas que la cuidan. - You are with people who care for you.

Usted está muy bien acompañada. - You are in very good company.

Practice Dialog

Respiremos juntos un momento. No hay prisa, yo le ayudo con lo que necesite.

No sé qué está pasando. ¿Por qué no puedo recordarlo?

Es normal sentirse así a veces. Está a salvo aquí conmigo. ¿Le gustaría que tomáramos un té tranquilos?

Sí, por favor. Eso suena bien. Gracias por su paciencia.

English translation:
Let's breathe together for a moment. There's no rush, I will help you with whatever you need.

I don't know what's happening. Why can't I remember?

It's normal to feel that way sometimes. You are safe here with me. Would you like for us to have some tea quietly?

Yes, please. That sounds good. Thank you for your patience.

Practice Scenario

La señora Rosa, agitada, buscaba a su esposo fallecido. Ana, su auxiliar de enfermería, se acercó calmadamente. "Estoy aquí, Rosa. Es de noche, estás segura en tu habitación". Le ofreció su medicamento para la ansiedad con un vaso de agua. Sostuvo su mano temblorosa y habló con suavidad hasta que la respiración de Rosa se calmó y se durmió.

English translation: Mrs. Rosa, agitated, was looking for her deceased husband. Ana, her nursing assistant, approached calmly. "I am here, Rosa. It's nighttime, you are safe in your room." She offered her anxiety medication with a glass of water.

She held her trembling hand and spoke softly until Rosa's breathing calmed and she fell asleep.

ENGAGING IN CONVERSATION AND ACTIVITIES

Key Vocabulary

Buenos días - BWEH-nos DEE-as - Good morning

¿Necesita ayuda? - neh-seh-SEE-tah ah-YOO-dah - Do you need help?

Vamos a tomar la medicina - VAH-mos ah toh-MAR lah meh-dee-SEE-nah - Let's take your medicine

¿Tiene dolor? - TYEH-neh doh-LOHR - Are you in pain?

¿Le ayudo a levantarse? - leh ah-YOO-doh ah leh-vahn-TAR-seh - Shall I help you get up?

Vamos a comer - VAH-mos ah koh-MEHR - Let's eat

¿Cómo amaneció? - KOH-moh ah-mah-neh-SYOH - How did you wake up? (How are you this morning?)

Señor / Señora - seh-NYOR / seh-NYOR-ah - Sir / Ma'am

Con cuidado - kohn kwee-DAH-doh - Carefully

¿Le gustaría...? - leh goos-tah-REE-ah - Would you like...?

¿Puede respirar hondo? - PWEH-deh rehs-pee-RAHR ON-doh - Can you take a deep breath?

Gracias - GRAH-syahs - Thank you

Grammatical Examples

¿Le gustaría tomar un paseo? - Would you like to take a walk?

¿Le gustaría escuchar música? - Would you like to listen to music?

¿Le gustaría ver fotografías? - Would you like to look at

photographs?

¿Le gustaría beber agua? - Would you like to drink some water?

¿Le gustaría jugar a las cartas? - Would you like to play cards?

Buenos días, ¿cómo amaneció hoy? ¿Le gustaría ayudarme a preparar el desayuno?

Muy bien, gracias por preguntar. Sí, me encantaría. Eso me hace sentir útil.

Perfecto. Juntos lo haremos. ¿Prefiere café o té hoy?

Té, por favor. Usted siempre es tan amable y paciente conmigo.

English translation:

Good morning, how did you wake up today? Would you like to help me prepare breakfast?

Very well, thank you for asking. Yes, I would love to. That makes me feel useful.

Perfect. We'll do it together. Do you prefer coffee or tea today?

Tea, please. You are always so kind and patient with me.

La Sra. García, con demencia avanzada, se resistía al baño. Ana, su auxiliar, le habló suavemente sobre su juventud mientras la ayudaba con la higiene personal. Usando una comunicación clara y respetuosa, Ana la vistió con su jersey favorito. Luego, compartieron un momento de compañerismo durante la merienda, fomentando su bienestar emocional.

English translation: Mrs. Garcia, with advanced dementia, resisted her bath. Ana, her aide, spoke softly to her about her youth while assisting with personal hygiene. Using clear and respectful communication, Ana dressed her in her favorite sweater. Then, they shared a moment of companionship during snack time, fostering her emotional well-being.

DEALING WITH DEMENTIA AND MEMORY ISSUES

¿Cómo está usted? - KOH-moh ehs-TAH oos-TEHD - How are you?

Vamos a ayudarle - VAH-mohs ah ah-yoo-DAHR-leh - We are going to help you

Es hora de su medicina - ehs OH-rah deh soo meh-dee-SEE-nah - It is time for your medicine

¿Le duele algo? - Leh DWEH-leh AHL-goh - Does something hurt you?

Vamos a bañarnos - VAH-mohs ah bah-NYAHR-nohs - Let's get bathed

¿Tiene hambre? - TYEH-neh AHM-breh - Are you hungry?

Aquí tiene agua - ah-KEE TYEH-neh AH-gwah - Here is some water

¿Necesita ir al baño? - Neh-seh-SEE-tah eer ahl BAH-nyoh - Do you need to use the bathroom?

Venga conmigo - VEHN-gah kohn-MEE-goh - Come with me

Descanse un poco - dehs-KAHN-seh oon POH-koh - Rest a little

Muy bien - MOO-ee byehn - Very good

Gracias - GRAH-syahs - Thank you

¿Recuerda usted su nombre? - Do you remember your name?

¿Recuerda usted dónde está su habitación? - Do you remember

where your room is?

¿Recuerda usted qué desayunó hoy? - Do you remember what you had for breakfast today?

¿Recuerda usted a su hijo? - Do you remember your son?

¿Recuerda usted tomar su medicina? - Do you remember to take your medicine?

Practice Dialog

Buenos días, ¿cómo amaneció hoy? Vamos a tomar el desayuno y luego sus pastillas.

¿Pastillas? ¿Yo tomo pastillas? No recuerdo haberlo hecho ayer.

Sí, señora, es su rutina de todas las mañanas. Le ayuda a mantenerse fuerte y sana.

Tiene razón, querida. A veces se me olvidan las cosas. Gracias por su paciencia.

English translation:

Good morning, how are you today? Let's have breakfast and then your pills.

Pills? I take pills? I don't remember doing that yesterday.

Yes, ma'am, it's your routine every morning. It helps you stay strong and healthy.

You're right, dear. Sometimes I forget things. Thank you for your patience.

Practice Scenario

La Sra. García repite la misma pregunta sobre el desayuno. Su auxiliar de enfermería, Ana, responde con paciencia mientras ayuda con la higiene personal. Después, revisan el tablero de orientación con la fecha y el clima. Ana utiliza frases cortas y mantiene contacto visual, validando los sentimientos de confusión de la residente sin corregirla. La rutina constante proporciona consuelo.

English translation:

Mrs. Garcia repeats the same question about breakfast. Her nursing assistant, Ana, responds patiently while assisting with personal hygiene. Later, they review the orientation board with the date and weather. Ana uses short phrases and maintains eye contact, validating the resident's feelings of confusion without correcting her. The constant routine provides comfort.

ENCOURAGING INDEPENDENCE AND DIGNITY

Key Vocabulary

¿Le gustaría intentarlo? - leh goos-tah-REE-ah een-ten-TAHR-loh - Would you like to try?

A su propio ritmo - ah soo PROH-pee-oh REET-moh - At your own pace

Usted puede hacerlo - oos-TED PWEH-deh ah-SER-loh - You can do it

¿Prefiere hacerlo solo/sola? - preh-fee-EH-reh ah-SER-loh SOH-loh / SOH-lah - Do you prefer to do it yourself?

Estoy aquí para ayudarle - es-TOY ah-KEE pah-rah ah-yoo-DAHR-leh - I am here to help you

Tómese su tiempo - TOH-meh-seh soo tee-EM-poh - Take your time

Muy bien - MOO-ee bee-EN - Very good

Excelente - ek-seh-LEN-teh - Excellent

¿Cómo le gustaría...? - KOH-moh leh goos-tah-REE-ah - How would you like...?

Es su decisión - es soo deh-see-see-OHN - It is your decision

¿Dónde le duele? - DOHN-deh leh DWEH-leh - Where does it hurt?

Vamos a... (bañarnos, vestirnos) - VAH-mohs ah (bahn-YAHR-nohs, ves-TEER-nohs) - Let's... (get bathed, get dressed)

Grammatical Examples

Usted puede elegir su ropa hoy. - You can choose your clothes today.

Usted puede caminar a su propio ritmo. - You can walk at your own pace.

Usted puede sostener su taza de café. - You can hold your coffee cup.

Usted puede decidir el menú para el almuerzo. - You can decide the menu for lunch.

Practice Dialog

Voy a ayudarle a vestirse, pero usted puede abrocharse los botones. Así practica.

Me gusta poder hacer algo yo solo. Me hace sentir útil.

Exactamente. Mantener su independencia es muy importante para su bienestar.

Gracias por su paciencia. Eso significa mucho para mí.

English translation:

I'm going to help you get dressed, but you can button the buttons. That way you practice.

I like being able to do something myself. It makes me feel useful.

Exactly. Maintaining your independence is very important for your well-being.

Thank you for your patience. That means a lot to me.

Practice Scenario

La Sra. García rechazó el baño. Ana, la auxiliar, no insistió. En cambio, ofreció elegir la ropa. "¿Prefiere el vestido azul o la blusa roja?". La Sra. García señaló la blusa. Ana le pasó las prendas, permitiéndole vestirse sola. Con paciencia, apoyó su autonomía, preservando su dignidad en cada pequeña decisión del cuidado diario.

English translation: Mrs. Garcia refused her bath. Ana, the aide, didn't insist. Instead, she offered a choice of clothes. "Do you prefer the blue dress or the red blouse?". Mrs. Garcia pointed to the blouse. Ana handed her the clothes, allowing her to dress herself. With patience, she supported her autonomy, preserving her dignity in every small daily care decision.

MANAGING BEHAVIORAL CHALLENGES

Key Vocabulary

¿Necesita ayuda? - neh-seh-SEE-tah ah-YOO-dah - Do you need help?

Vamos a tomar la medicina - VAH-mohs ah toh-MAHR lah meh-dee-SEE-nah - Let's take your medicine

¿Tiene dolor? - TYEH-neh doh-LOHR - Are you in pain?

Por favor, siéntese - pohr fah-VOHR, see-EN-teh-seh - Please, sit down

Respire profundamente - rehs-PEE-reh proh-foon-dah-MEN-teh - Breathe deeply

Estoy aquí para ayudarle - ehs-TOY ah-KEE pah-rah ah-yoo-DAHR-leh - I am here to help you

¿Puede esperar un momento? - PWEH-deh ehs-peh-RAHR oon moh-MEN-toh - Can you wait a moment?

Tranquilo/a - trahn-KEE-loh/lah - Calm (said reassuringly)

Vamos a caminar despacio - VAH-mohs ah kah-mee-NAHR dehs-PAH-syoh - Let's walk slowly

¿Le molesta algo? - Leh moh-LEHS-tah AHL-goh - Is something bothering you?

Es hora de descansar - ehs OH-rah deh dehs-kahn-SAHR - It's time to rest

Gracias por su cooperación - GRAH-syahs pohr soo koh-oh-peh-rah-SYOHN - Thank you for your cooperation

Grammatical Examples

El señor necesita calma - The gentleman needs calmness.

La señora necesita calma - The lady needs calmness.

El residente necesita calma - The resident (male) needs calmness.

La residente necesita calma - The resident (female) needs calmness.

El paciente necesita calma - The patient (male) needs calmness.

La paciente necesita calma - The patient (female) needs calmness.

Practice Dialog

Entiendo que esté frustrado, pero por su seguridad necesito que me deje ayudarle a levantarse.

No quiero ayuda, puedo hacerlo yo solo. Déjeme en paz.

Le prometo que lo haré con cuidado. Vamos a intentarlo juntos, paso a paso.

…Está bien. Pero despacio, por favor.

English translation:

I understand you're frustrated, but for your safety I need you to let me help you get up.

I don't want help, I can do it myself. Leave me alone.

I promise I will do it carefully. Let's try it together, step by step.

…Okay. But slowly, please.

Practice Scenario

La Sra. García, con demencia, se agitaba durante el baño. La auxiliar, Carmen, usó un tono calmado y le explicó cada paso. Le ofreció una toalla tibia para sus manos, distrayéndola. Carmen validó sus feelings diciendo: "Sé que esto es molesto". La Sra. García se calmó, permitiendo el aseo con dignidad.

English translation:

Mrs. Garcia, with dementia, became agitated during her bath. The aide, Carmen, used a calm tone and explained each step.

She offered a warm towel for her hands, distracting her. Carmen validated her feelings by saying, "I know this is bothersome." Mrs. Garcia calmed down, allowing the hygiene care with dignity.

CALLING FOR MEDICAL HELP

¿Necesita ayuda? - neh-seh-SEE-tah ah-YOO-dah - Do you need help?

Llame al 911 - YAH-meh ahl noh-veh-see-EH-zohs - Call 911

Emergencia - eh-mehr-HEN-syah - Emergency

¿Dónde le duele? - DOHN-deh leh doo-EH-leh - Where does it hurt?

Señor/Señora - seh-NYOR/seh-NYOR-ah - Sir/Ma'am

Respire profundamente - rehs-PEE-reh proh-foon-dah-MEN-teh - Breathe deeply

¿Puede hablar? - PWEH-deh ah-BLAR - Can you speak?

Ataque al corazón - ah-TAH-keh ahl koh-rah-SOHN - Heart attack

Caída - kah-EE-dah - Fall

Ambulancia - ahm-boo-LAN-syah - Ambulancy

No se mueva - noh seh MWEH-vah - Don't move

Estoy aquí para ayudarle - ehs-TOY ah-KEE pah-rah ah-yoo-DAR-leh - I am here to help you

Grammatical Examples

Necesito una ambulancia para un señor mayor. - I need an ambulance for an elderly gentleman.

Necesito una ambulancia para una señora mayor. - I need an ambulance for an elderly lady.

Necesito una ambulancia para un paciente. - I need an ambulance for a male patient.

Necesito una ambulancia para una paciente. - I need an ambulance for a female patient.

Necesito una ambulancia para un residente. - I need an ambulance for a male resident.

Necesito una ambulancia para una residente. - I need an ambulance for a female resident.

Practice Dialog

Señora, ¿se siente bien? Veo que está muy pálida y le cuesta respirar.

No, no me siento bien. Tengo un dolor muy fuerte en el pecho.

Voy a llamar al 911 de inmediato. Por favor, trate de mantenerse tranquila mientras hablo con ellos.

Gracias. ¿Podría tomar mi mano, por favor?

Practice Scenario

La auxiliar Rosa notó que don Carlos respiraba con dificultad. Rápidamente, usó el botón de llamada para alertar a la enfermera. Mientras llegaba la ayuda, Rosa lo tranquilizó, le tomó los signos vitales y preparó su historial médico. Mantuvo la calma para asegurar una respuesta rápida y un traslado eficiente al hospital.

English translation:

The aide Rosa noticed Mr. Carlos was breathing with difficulty. She quickly used the call button to alert the nurse. While help arrived, Rosa reassured him, took his vital signs, and prepared his medical history. She remained calm to ensure a quick response and an efficient transfer to the hospital.

FALL RESPONSE AND INJURY ASSESSMENT

Key Vocabulary

¿Se cayó? - seh kah-YOH - Did you fall?

¿Dónde le duele? - DOHN-deh leh doo-EH-leh - Where does it hurt?

Voy a ayudarle - voy ah ah-yoo-DAHR-leh - I am going to help you

Necesito revisarle - neh-seh-SEE-toh reh-bee-SAHR-leh - I need to check you

¿Puede mover...? - PWEH-deh moh-BEHR - Can you move...?

¿Qué pasó? - keh pah-SOH - What happened?

Respire hondo - rehs-PEE-reh ON-doh - Take a deep breath

Despacio, por favor - dehs-PAH-syoh pohr fah-BOHR - Slowly, please

Señor/Señora - seh-NYOR/seh-NYOH-rah - Sir/Ma'am

Vamos a sentarnos - VAH-mohs ah sen-TAHR-nohs - Let's sit down

¿Necesita su medicamento? - neh-seh-SEE-tah soo meh-dee-kah-MEN-toh - Do you need your medicine?

¿Tiene mareos? - TYEH-neh mah-REH-ohs - Are you dizzy?

Grammatical Examples

¿Le duele el brazo? - Does your arm hurt?

¿Le duele la pierna? - Does your leg hurt?

¿Le duele la cabeza? - Does your head hurt?

¿Le duele la espalda? - Does your back hurt?

¿Le duele el hombro? - Does your shoulder hurt?

¿Le duele la cadera? - Does your hip hurt?

Practice Dialog

¿Señora, ¿está bien? ¿Puede decirme qué pasó?

Me resbalé y me caí. Me duele mucho la muñeca.

Voy a llamar a la enfermera. Por favor, no se mueva. ¿Le duele en algún otro lugar?

Solo la muñeca. Ay, duele mucho al moverla.

English translation:

Ma'am, are you okay? Can you tell me what happened?

I slipped and fell. My wrist hurts a lot.

I'm going to call the nurse. Please, don't move. Does it hurt anywhere else?

Just the wrist. Oh, it hurts a lot to move it.

Practice Scenario

La señora Rodríguez se resbaló en el baño. La auxiliar, Elena, no la movió. Calmadamente, evaluó su estado mental y le preguntó por el dolor. Observó si había deformidad o hinchazón en su cadera y hombro. Luego, reportó el incidente al enfermero, detallando los hallazgos antes de cualquier movilización, asegurando una respuesta segura y protocolos de prevención de caídas.

English translation: Mrs. Rodriguez slipped in the bathroom. The aide, Elena, did not move her. Calmly, she assessed her mental state and asked about pain. She looked for deformity or swelling in her hip and shoulder. Then, she reported the incident to the nurse, detailing the findings before any movement, ensuring a safe response and fall prevention protocols.

CHOKING ASSISTANCE AND FIRST AID

¿Se está ahogando? - seh ehs-TAH ah-oh-GAHN-doh - Are you choking?

Tosa fuerte - TOH-sah FWEHR-teh - Cough hard

No puedo respirar - noh PWEH-doh rehs-pee-RAHR - I can't breathe

Ayúdeme, por favor - ah-YOO-deh-meh pohr fah-VOHR - Help me, please

Incline la cabeza hacia adelante - een-KLEE-neh lah kah-BEH-sah AH-see-ah ah-deh-LAHN-teh - Tilt your head forward

Abra la boca - AH-brah lah BOH-kah - Open your mouth

Voy a ayudarle - voy ah ah-yoo-DAHR-leh - I am going to help you

¿Puede toser? - PWEH-deh toh-SEHR - Can you cough?

Está bien, respire despacio - ehs-TAH bee-EHN rehs-PEE-reh dehs-PAH-see-oh - It's okay, breathe slowly

Necesito llamar a la enfermera - neh-seh-SEE-toh yah-MAHR ah lah ehn-fehr-MEH-rah - I need to call the nurse

¿Puede hablar? - PWEH-deh ah-BLAHR - Can you speak?

Quédese tranquilo/a - KEH-deh-seh trahn-KEE-loh/lah - Stay calm

Señora, ¿se está ahogando? - Ma'am, are you choking?

Señor, ¿se está ahogando? - Sir, are you choking?
¿Se está ahogando, doña Elena? - Are you choking, Doña Elena?
¿Se está ahogando, don Carlos? - Are you choking, Don Carlos?

Practice Dialog

¿Señora, ¿puede toser o está ahogándose? ¡Necesito que me conteste!
(Agitando la cabeza, agarrando su garganta)

¡Voy a aplicar compresiones abdominales! Esto la ayudará.
(Colocándose detrás de la persona)

Una, dos, tres… ¿Salió? ¿Ya puede respirar?
(Suelta un objeto y jadea)

Muy bien, respire despacio. Ahora la revisaré y llamaremos al médico.

Practice Scenario

La residente comenzó a ahogarse con un pedazo de pan. Inmediatamente, la auxiliar de enfermería realizó la maniobra de Heimlich desde atrás. Tras dos compresiones, la obstrucción se desalojó. La auxiliar calmó a la señora, le ofreció agua y verificó su oxigenación con el pulsioxímetro. Documentó el incidente en el informe de turno para supervisión.

English translation:
The resident began to choke on a piece of bread. Immediately, the nursing assistant performed the Heimlich maneuver from behind. After two compressions, the obstruction was dislodged. The aide calmed the woman, offered her water, and verified her oxygenation with the pulse oximeter. She documented the incident in the shift report for supervision.

RECOGNIZING STROKE OR HEART ATTACK SYMPTOMS

Key Vocabulary

¿Se siente bien? - seh see-EN-teh bee-EN - Do you feel well?

Dolor en el pecho - doh-LOHR en el PEH-choh - Pain in the chest

¿Tiene dificultad para respirar? - tee-EH-neh dee-fee-kool-TAHD PAH-rah res-pee-RAHR - Do you have difficulty breathing?

Mareado/Mareada - mah-reh-AH-doh/mah-reh-AH-dah - Dizzy (male/female)

Entumecimiento - en-too-meh-see-mee-EN-toh - Numbness

Debilidad - deh-bee-lee-DAHD - Weakness

¿Puede sonreír? - PWEH-deh son-reh-EER - Can you smile?

¿Puede levantar ambos brazos? - PWEH-deh leh-vahn-TAHR AHM-bohs BRAH-sohs - Can you raise both arms?

¿Puede hablar claramente? - PWEH-deh ah-BLAHR klah-rah-MEN-teh - Can you speak clearly?

Confusión - kohn-foo-see-OHN - Confusion

Dolor de cabeza fuerte - doh-LOHR deh kah-BEH-sah FWEHR-teh - Strong headache

Llame al nueve-uno-uno - YAH-meh ahl NWEH-beh OO-noh OO-noh - Call nine-one-one

Grammatical Examples

Él tiene dolor en el pecho. - He has chest pain.

Ella tiene dolor en el pecho. - She has chest pain.

Usted tiene dolor en el pecho. - You (formal) have chest pain.

La señora tiene dolor en el pecho. - The lady has chest pain.
El señor tiene dolor en el pecho. - The gentleman has chest pain.

Practice Dialog

¿Señora, se siente bien? Su cara se ve un poco caída y su habla es confusa.

Ay, sí, es que tengo un dolor de cabeza horrible y me siento muy débil del lado derecho.

Necesito llamar a los servicios de emergencia de inmediato. Estos pueden ser síntomas de un derrame cerebral.

Por favor, hágalo. Me está dando mucho miedo.

English translation:

Ma'am, are you feeling okay? Your face looks a little droopy and your speech is slurred.

Oh, yes, it's just that I have a terrible headache and I feel very weak on my right side.

I need to call emergency services right away. These could be symptoms of a stroke.

Please, do it. I'm getting very scared.

Practice Scenario

La señora Rosa, usuaria de cuidados domiciliarios, comenzó a hablar con dificultad y mostró debilidad en un lado del cuerpo. Su auxiliar de enfermería, reconociendo los signos de un accidente cerebrovascular, activó inmediatamente el protocolo de emergencia. Mantuvo la calma, aseguró a la señora Rosa y llamó al servicio de urgencias, salvando así una vida con su observación diligente.

English translation:

Mrs. Rosa, a home care user, began to speak with difficulty and showed weakness on one side of her body. Her nursing aide, recognizing the signs of a stroke, immediately activated the emergency protocol. She remained calm, reassured Mrs. Rosa, and called the emergency service, thus saving a life with her diligent observation.

CONTACTING FAMILY IN EMERGENCIES

Key Vocabulary

¿Necesita ayuda? - neh-seh-SEE-tah ah-YOO-dah - Do you need help?

¿Dónde le duele? - DOHN-deh leh doo-EH-leh - Where does it hurt?

Voy a llamar a su familia - voy ah yah-MAHR ah soo fah-MEE-lee-ah - I am going to call your family

Su hijo/hija está en camino - soo EE-hoh / EE-hah ehs-TAH ehn kah-MEE-noh - Your son/daughter is on the way

¿Puede respirar profundamente? - PWEH-deh rehs-pee-RAHR proh-foon-dah-MEN-teh - Can you breathe deeply?

Tenemos que ir al hospital - teh-NEH-mohs keh eer ahl ohs-pee-TAHL - We have to go to the hospital

¿Tiene sus medicamentos? - tee-EH-neh soos meh-dee-kah-MEN-tohs - Do you have your medications?

Abuelito/Abuelita - ah-bweh-LEE-toh / ah-bweh-LEE-tah - Grandfather/Grandmother (affectionate, respectful)

Está todo bien - ehs-TAH TOH-doh bee-EN - Everything is okay

¿Puede tomar agua? - PWEH-deh toh-MAHR AH-gwah - Can you drink some water?

Vamos a ayudarle - VAH-mohs ah ah-yoo-DAHR-leh - We are going to help you

¿Cuál es el número de su familiar? - KWAHL ehs ehl NOO-meh-roh deh soo fah-mee-lee-AHR - What is your family member's number?

Su hijo necesita venir ahora. - Your son needs to come now.

Su hija necesita venir ahora. - Your daughter needs to come now.

Sus hijos necesitan venir ahora. - Your children (sons) need to come now.

Sus hijas necesitan venir ahora. - Your daughters need to come now.

Practice Dialog

¿Señora, puedo ayudarla a llamar a su hija para contarle lo sucedido?

Sí, por favor. ¿Podría decirle que estoy bien, pero que vamos al hospital?

Por supuesto. También le diré qué hospital y le pediré que se reúna con nosotros allí.

Gracias. Me quedo más tranquila sabiendo que ella lo sabe.

English translation:

Ma'am, can I help you call your daughter to tell her what happened?

Yes, please. Could you tell her I'm fine, but that we're going to the hospital?

Of course. I will also tell her which hospital and ask her to meet us there.

Thank you. I feel better knowing that she knows.

Practice Scenario

La señora Rosa, con demencia avanzada, se agitó. La auxiliar de enfermería verificó sus signos vitales y calmó la situación. Siguiendo el protocolo, contactó a su hija usando la lista de números de emergencia. Documentó el incidente en el informe de turno, asegurando una comunicación clara entre el equipo de cuidadores y la familia para el bienestar de la residente.

English translation:

Mrs. Rosa, with advanced dementia, became agitated. The

nursing assistant verified her vital signs and calmed the situation. Following protocol, she contacted her daughter using the list of emergency numbers. She documented the incident in the shift report, ensuring clear communication between the caregiving team and the family for the resident's well-being.

HOUSEHOLD TASKS AND LIGHT CLEANING

¿Le ayudo a levantarse? - leh ah-YOO-doh ah leh-vahn-TAHR-seh - May I help you get up?

Vamos a bañarnos - VAH-mohs ah bah-NYAHR-nohs - Let's bathe ourselves

¿Necesita usar el baño? - neh-seh-SEE-tah oo-SAHR ehl BAH-nyoh - Do you need to use the bathroom?

Voy a limpiar la habitación - voy ah leem-pee-AHR lah ah-bee-tah-see-OHN - I am going to clean the room

¿Tiene hambre? - tee-EH-neh AHM-breh - Are you hungry?

Voy a cambiar las sábanas - voy ah kahm-bee-AHR lahs SAH-bah-nahs - I am going to change the sheets

Es hora de comer - ehs OH-rah deh koh-MEHR - It's time to eat

Tome su medicina - TOH-meh soo meh-dee-SEE-nah - Take your medicine

¿Está cómodo/a? - ehs-TAH KOH-moh-doh/dah - Are you comfortable?

Vamos a vestirnos - VAH-mohs ah vehs-TEER-nohs - Let's get dressed

Permítame ayudarle - pehr-MEE-tah-meh ah-yoo-DAHR-leh - Allow me to help you

¿Le duele algo? - leh doo-EH-leh AHL-goh - Does anything hurt you?

Grammatical Examples

Voy a limpiar la habitación ahora. - I am going to clean the room now.

Vas a limpiar la habitación ahora. - You are going to clean the room now.

Va a limpiar la habitación ahora. - You (formal) are going to clean the room now.

Vamos a limpiar la habitación ahora. - We are going to clean the room now.

Van a limpiar la habitación ahora. - They are going to clean the room now.

Practice Dialog

¿Le gustaría que pasemos la aspiradora en la sala hoy? Hace bastante polvo.

Sí, por favor. Después, ¿podría ayudarme a doblar esa pila de ropa limpia?

Por supuesto. Primero terminemos aquí y luego la organizamos juntos.

Muchas gracias. Hacer estas tareas con compañía es mucho más agradable.

English translation:

Would you like us to vacuum the living room today? It's quite dusty.

Yes, please. Afterwards, could you help me fold that pile of clean laundry?

Of course. Let's finish here first and then we'll organize it together.

Thank you very much. Doing these tasks with company is much more pleasant.

Practice Scenario

La auxiliar Rosa ayuda a la señora Elena con el aseo matutino. Le lava la cara con una toallita tibia y le cepilla el cabello suavemente. Luego, Rosa cambia las sábanas de la cama con cuidado mientras Elena descansa en su sillón. Después de ordenar la habitación, asegura que el caminador esté cerca para movilizarse de forma segura.

English translation:
The aide Rosa helps Mrs. Elena with her morning hygiene. She washes her face with a warm washcloth and brushes her hair gently. Then, Rosa changes the bed sheets carefully while Elena rests in her chair. After tidying the room, she ensures the walker is nearby for safe mobility.

LAUNDRY AND CLOTHING CARE

Lavar la ropa - lah-BAHR lah ROH-pah - To wash the clothes

¿Le ayudo a cambiarse? - leh ah-YOO-doh ah kahm-bee-AHR-seh - May I help you change?

Su pijama - soo pee-HAH-mah - Your pajamas

Ropa limpia - ROH-pah LEEM-pee-ah - Clean clothes

Ropa sucia - ROH-pah SOO-see-ah - Dirty clothes

¿Está cómodo/a? - ehs-TAH KOH-moh-doh/dah - Are you comfortable?

Vamos a vestirnos - VAH-mohs ah vehs-TEER-nohs - Let's get dressed

¿Prefiere esta camisa? - preh-fee-EH-reh EHS-tah kah-MEE-sah - Do you prefer this shirt?

Los calcetines - lohs kahl-seh-TEE-nehs - The socks

¿Tiene frío? - tee-EH-neh FREE-oh - Are you cold?

¿Tiene calor? - tee-EH-neh kah-LOHR - Are you warm?

La lavadora - lah lah-bah-DOH-rah - The washing machine

Lavo la ropa blanca con agua caliente. - I wash the white clothes with hot water.

Lavo la ropa de color con agua fría. - I wash the colored clothes with cold water.

Lavo las sábanas sucias. - I wash the dirty sheets.

Lavo las toallas húmedas. - I wash the damp towels.

Lavo la bata favorita del señor García. - I wash Mr. Garcia's favorite robe.

Lavo la ropa delicada a mano. - I wash the delicate clothes by hand.

Practice Dialog

¿Señora, prefiere que lave esta blusa a mano o puedo meterla en la lavadora con el resto de la ropa?

Prefiero que la laves a mano, por favor. Es muy especial para mí.

Por supuesto. La lavaré con agua fría y un jabón suave para protegerla.

Muchas gracias, cariño. Usted siempre es tan cuidadosa con mis cosas.

English translation:

Ma'am, would you prefer I wash this blouse by hand or can I put it in the washing machine with the rest of the clothes?

I prefer you wash it by hand, please. It is very special to me.

Of course. I will wash it in cold water with a mild soap to protect it.

Thank you very much, dear. You are always so careful with my things.

Practice Scenario

La señora Rosa observa mientras su auxiliar dobla su suéter favorito. "Usé agua fría y jabón suave para proteger la tela", explica la auxiliar. Revisa las etiquetas de cuidado antes de lavar, separando la ropa delicada. Coloca la ropa limpia en el cajón, manteniendo el orden que a la señora Rosa le gusta. Este cuidado meticuloso preserva su dignidad y comodidad diaria.

English translation: Mrs. Rosa watches as her aide folds her favorite sweater. "I used cold water and mild soap to protect the fabric," the aide explains. She checks the care labels before washing, separating the delicate clothing. She places the clean clothes in the drawer, maintaining the order Mrs. Rosa likes. This meticulous care preserves her dignity and daily comfort.

TRANSPORTATION TO APPOINTMENTS

Key Vocabulary

¿Está listo/a para ir? - EHS-tah LEES-toh/ah pah-rah eer - Are you ready to go?

Vamos a su cita - VAH-mohs ah soo SEE-tah - We are going to your appointment

El coche está aquí - el KOH-cheh ehs-tah ah-KEE - The car is here

Necesito ayudarle a subir - neh-seh-SEE-toh ah-yoo-DAHR-leh ah soo-BEER - I need to help you get in

Por favor, póngase el cinturón de seguridad - pohr fah-VOHR, POHN-gah-seh el seen-too-ROHN deh seh-goo-ree-DAHD - Please put on your seatbelt

Con cuidado - kohn kwee-DAH-doh - Carefully

¿Se siente cómodo/a? - seh see-EN-teh KOH-moh-doh/dah - Do you feel comfortable?

Tranquilo/a - trahn-KEE-loh/lah - Don't worry / Be calm

Llegamos - yeh-GAH-mohs - We have arrived

Necesito la silla de ruedas - neh-seh-SEE-toh lah SEE-yah deh RWEH-dahs - I need the wheelchair

Espera un momento - ehs-PEH-rah oon moh-MEN-toh - Wait a moment

Vamos a entrar - VAH-mohs ah ehn-TRAHR - Let's go inside

Grammatical Examples

El señor necesita ir al médico. - The gentleman needs to go to the doctor.

La señora necesita ir al hospital. - The lady needs to go to the hospital.

El paciente necesita ir a terapia. - The patient needs to go to therapy.

La residente necesita ir a la farmacia. - The resident needs to go to the pharmacy.

Practice Dialog

Buenos días, señora. ¿Está lista para su cita con el cardiólogo?

Sí, gracias. ¿Podría traer mi andador, por favor?

Por supuesto, aquí está. Vamos a ir despacio, no hay prisa.

Muy bien. Le agradezco su paciencia.

Practice Scenario

La señora Rosa espera en su silla de ruedas para su cita médica. Su auxiliar, Elena, verifica su medicación y la abrocha con el cinturón de seguridad en la furgoneta. Durante el trayecto, Elena le habla con calma para minimizar su ansiedad. Llegan puntuales al consultorio, listos para el chequeo de rutina de la señora Rosa.

English translation: Mrs. Rosa waits in her wheelchair for her medical appointment. Her aide, Elena, checks her medication and fastens her seatbelt in the van. During the trip, Elena speaks to her calmly to minimize her anxiety. They arrive on time at the doctor's office, ready for Mrs. Rosa's routine checkup.

SHOPPING AND ERRANDS

¿Necesita ayuda? - neh-seh-SEE-tah ah-YOO-dah - Do you need help?

Vamos de compras - VAH-mohs deh KOHM-prahs - We are going shopping

La lista - lah LEES-tah - The list

El supermercado - el soo-pehr-mehr-KAH-doh - The supermarket

La farmacia - lah fahr-MAH-syah - The pharmacy

¿Qué le gustaría comer? - keh leh goos-tah-REE-ah koh-MEHR - What would you like to eat?

Es hora de su medicina - ehs OH-rah deh soo meh-dee-SEE-nah - It is time for your medicine

¿Tiene dolor? - TYEH-neh doh-LOHR - Are you in pain?

¿Le ayudo a pagar? - leh ah-YOO-doh ah pah-GAHR - Shall I help you pay?

Respetado señor - rehs-peh-TAH-doh seh-NYOHR - Respected sir
Respetada señora - rehs-peh-TAH-dah seh-NYOH-rah - Respected madam

¿Está cómodo/a? - ehs-TAH KOH-moh-doh/dah - Are you comfortable?

Grammatical Examples

¿Necesita usted la medicina? - Do you need the medicine?
¿Necesita usted los zapatos? - Do you need the shoes?
¿Necesita usted las revistas? - Do you need the magazines?

¿Necesita usted el pan? - Do you need the bread?

Practice Dialog

Buenos días, ¿necesita que le compre algo de la farmacia o del supermercado hoy?

Sí, por favor. Necesito mi crema para la piel y pan integral.

Perfecto. Apunto la crema hidratante sin perfume y el pan integral. ¿Algo más?

No, eso es todo. Muchas gracias por su ayuda.

English translation:

Good morning, do you need me to buy something from the pharmacy or the supermarket for you today?

Yes, please. I need my skin cream and whole wheat bread.

Perfect. I'll write down the fragrance-free moisturizing cream and the whole wheat bread. Anything else?

No, that's all. Thank you very much for your help.

Practice Scenario

La Sra. García revisa su lista de compras. Su auxiliar, Elena, le ayuda a recordar los artículos. En la tienda, Elena empuja la silla de ruedas mientras la Sra. García elige el champú y las galletas. De regreso, organizan los medicamentos y los suministros en el estante. La Sra. García sonríe, agradecida por la compañía y la ayuda con sus quehaceres.

English translation: Mrs. Garcia reviews her shopping list. Her aide, Elena, helps her remember the items. In the store, Elena pushes the wheelchair while Mrs. Garcia chooses the shampoo and cookies. Back home, they organize the medications and supplies on the shelf. Mrs. Garcia smiles, grateful for the company and help with her errands.

MANAGING FINANCES AND BILLS

Key Vocabulary

¿Necesita ayuda con las facturas? - neh-seh-SEE-tah ah-YOO-dah kohn lahs fahk-TOO-rahs - Do you need help with the bills?

El pago de la renta - ehl PAH-goh deh lah REHN-tah - The rent payment

La cuenta de electricidad - lah KWEHN-tah deh eh-lek-tree-see-DAHD - The electricity bill

Presupuesto mensual - preh-soo-PWEHS-toh mehn-SWAHL - Monthly budget

¿Dónde guarda los estados de cuenta? - DOHN-deh GWAHR-dah lohs ehs-TAH-dohs deh KWEHN-tah - Where do you keep the account statements?

Su pensión - soo pehn-see-OHN - Your pension

¿Pudó firmar el cheque? - poo-DOH feer-MAHR ehl CHEH-keh - Were you able to sign the check?

Gastos de la casa - GAHS-tohs deh lah KAH-sah - Household expenses

Dinero para el supermercado - dee-NEH-roh PAH-rah ehl soo-pehr-mehr-KAH-doh - Money for the supermarket

Tarjeta de débito - tar-HEH-tah deh DEH-bee-toh - Debit card

¿Le gustaría que revisemos juntos? - leh goos-tah-REE-ah keh reh-bee-SEH-mohs HOON-tohs - Would you like us to review it together?

Es importante pagar a tiempo - ehs eem-pohr-TAHN-teh pah-GAHR ah tee-EHM-poh - It is important to pay on time

Grammatical Examples

Usted necesita pagar la factura del agua. - You need to pay the water bill.

Usted debe revisar el estado de cuenta. - You should review the bank statement.

Usted tiene que firmar el cheque. - You have to sign the check.

Usted puede organizar los recibos. - You can organize the receipts.

Usted debe guardar los documentos importantes. - You must keep the important documents.

Practice Dialog

¿Señora, ya pagamos el recibo de la luz en línea. ¿Le gustaría que revisemos juntos el estado de cuenta bancario ahora?

Sí, por favor. A veces me confundo con estos números nuevos. Agradezco su ayuda.

Claro que sí. Mire, aquí está el depósito de su pensión y estos son los pagos programados. Todo está en orden.

Muchas gracias. Me quedo más tranquila sabiendo que todo está al día.

English translation:
Ma'am, we've already paid the electricity bill online. Would you like us to review the bank statement together now?

Yes, please. I sometimes get confused with these new numbers. I appreciate your help.

Of course. Look, here is your pension deposit and these are the scheduled payments. Everything is in order.

Thank you so much. I feel more at ease knowing everything is up to date.

Practice Scenario

La señora Eva olvidó pagar la luz. Su auxiliar, Ana, revisó con ella el estado de cuentas. Juntas organizaron las facturas por fecha de vencimiento. Ana le recordó amablemente el pago programado en línea, asegurándose de que Eva entendiera y aprobara cada transacción para mantener su autonomía y la seguridad de su hogar de adultos mayores.

English translation:
Mrs. Eva forgot to pay the electricity bill. Her aide, Ana, reviewed the account statements with her. Together they organized the bills by due date. Ana kindly reminded her of the scheduled online payment, ensuring Eva understood and approved each transaction to maintain her autonomy and the security of her senior living home.

PROVIDING COMFORT CARE AND PAIN RELIEF

¿Cómo se siente hoy? - KOH-moh seh SYEN-teh oy - How are you feeling today?

Voy a ayudarle - voy ah ah-yoo-DAHR-leh - I am going to help you

¿Le duele aquí? - leh DWEH-leh ah-KEE - Does it hurt here?

Vamos a moverle con cuidado - VAH-mohs ah moh-BEHR-leh kohn kwhy-DAH-doh - We are going to move you carefully

Tome su medicina - TOH-meh soo meh-dee-SEE-nah - Take your medicine

Está bien, descanse - ehs-TAH byen, dehs-KAHN-seh - It's okay, rest

¿Necesita algo más? - neh-seh-SEE-tah AHL-goh mahs - Do you need anything else?

Voy a traerle agua - voy ah trah-EHR-leh AH-gwah - I will bring you some water

¿Está cómodo/a? - ehs-TAH KOH-moh-doh/dah - Are you comfortable?

Respire profundamente - rehs-PEE-reh proh-foon-dah-MEN-teh - Breathe deeply

Un momento, por favor - oon moh-MEN-toh pohr fah-VOHR - One moment, please

¿Así está mejor? - ah-SEE ehs-TAH meh-HOHR - Is that better?

135

Grammatical Examples

Le doy su medicina para el dolor. - I give you your pain medicine.

Le ayudo a sentarse cómodamente. - I help you sit comfortably.

Le preparo una compresa tibia. - I prepare a warm compress for you.

Le leo un libro para relajarse. - I read a book to you to relax.

Le arreglo las almohadas para su espalda. - I adjust the pillows for your back.

Le traigo una manta para que tenga calor. - I bring you a blanket so you are warm.

Practice Dialog

Voy a ajustar la almohada y le traigo el medicamento para el dolor, ¿le parece bien?

Sí, por favor. La molestia en la espalda no me deja descansar.

Aquí está. Con esto se sentirá más cómodo y podrá dormir mejor.

Muchas gracias. Se siente un poco de alivio ya.

English translation:

I'm going to adjust your pillow and bring you your pain medication, does that sound good?

Yes, please. The discomfort in my back won't let me rest.

Here you go. This will help you feel more comfortable and sleep better.

Thank you very much. I feel a little relief already.

Practice Scenario

La Sra. García, postrada en cama, gemía. La auxiliar de enfermería, Elena, le ofreció el analgésico según lo pautado. Luego, con suaves movimientos, le aplicó crema hidratante en la espalda seca y la cambió de posición con una almohada de apoyo. Le habló con calma, asegurándose de que estuviera cómoda y segura. Los gemidos cesaron, reemplazados por una respiración tranquila.

English translation: Mrs. García, bedridden, moaned. The

nursing assistant, Elena, offered her the painkiller as prescribed. Then, with gentle movements, she applied moisturizing cream to her dry back and repositioned her with a support pillow. She spoke calmly, ensuring she was comfortable and safe. The moans ceased, replaced by calm breathing.

COMMUNICATING WITH HOSPICE TEAMS

Key Vocabulary

¿Cómo se siente hoy? - KOH-moh seh see-EN-teh oy - How do you feel today?

¿Necesita ayuda para ir al baño? - neh-seh-SEE-tah ah-YOO-dah pah-rah eer ahl BAH-nyoh - Do you need help going to the bathroom?

Voy a tomar su temperatura. - voy ah toh-MAHR soo tem-peh-rah-TOO-rah - I am going to take your temperature.

Voy a cambiar su pañal. - voy ah kahm-bee-AIR soo pah-NYAHL - I am going to change your diaper.

¿Tiene dolor? - tee-EH-neh doh-LOHR - Are you in pain?

Vamos a sentarle. - VAH-mohs ah sen-TAR-leh - Let's sit you up.

Es hora de su medicina. - es OH-rah deh soo meh-dee-SEE-nah - It's time for your medicine.

¿Tiene sed? - tee-EH-neh sed - Are you thirsty?

¿Le aprieta el oxígeno? - leh ah-pree-EH-tah el ohk-SEE-heh-noh - Is the oxygen too tight?

Voy a acomodarle la almohada. - voy ah ah-koh-moh-DAR-leh lah ahl-moh-AH-dah - I am going to adjust your pillow.

¿Le gustaría un masaje? - leh goos-tah-REE-ah oon mah-SAH-heh - Would you like a massage?

Descance, estoy aquí con usted. - des-KAN-seh, es-TOY ah-KEE con oos-TED - Rest, I am here with you.

Grammatical Examples

¿Necesita usted más medicamento para el dolor? - Do you need more pain medication?

¿Necesita el señor más medicamento para el dolor? - Does sir need more pain medication?

¿Necesita la señora más medicamento para el dolor? - Does ma'am need more pain medication?

¿Necesita el paciente una manta adicional? - Does the patient need an extra blanket?

¿Necesita la paciente una manta adicional? - Does the patient need an extra blanket?

Practice Dialog

¿Noté que hoy no ha querido tomar los líquidos. ¿Le gustaría intentar con un heladito de agua?

Sí, por favor. Eso suena bien. A veces es más fácil de tomar así.

Perfecto. Se lo traigo en un momentito. También voy a anotarlo en su plan de cuidado para que todos lo sepamos.

Gracias. Se preocupan mucho por su comodidad.

English translation:

I noticed he hasn't wanted to drink any liquids today. Would you like to try some water ice?

Yes, please. That sounds good. Sometimes it's easier to take it that way.

Perfect. I'll bring it to you in just a moment. I'll also note it in his care plan so everyone is aware.

Thank you. You all care a lot about his comfort.

Practice Scenario

La auxiliar Rosa notó que el señor López, normalmente tranquilo, estaba agitado. Siguiendo el protocolo, documentó los cambios en su estado y reportó inmediatamente al equipo de hospice. La enfermera evaluó y ajustó su plan de cuidados, enfocándose en su confort. Rosa implementó las nuevas pautas de comunicación no verbal, asegurando su bienestar con compasión y profesionalismo.

English translation: The aide Rosa noticed that Mr.

Lopez, normally calm, was agitated. Following protocol, she documented the changes in his condition and reported immediately to the hospice team. The nurse assessed and adjusted his care plan, focusing on his comfort. Rosa implemented the new non-verbal communication guidelines, ensuring his well-being with compassion and professionalism.

SUPPORTING GRIEVING FAMILY MEMBERS

Lo siento mucho - loh see-EN-toh MOO-choh - I am so sorry

Acompañarlo/a en este momento - ah-kom-pahn-YAR-loh/lah en ES-teh mo-MEN-toh - To accompany you in this moment

¿Necesita un momento a solas? - neh-seh-SEE-tah oon mo-MEN-toh ah SOH-las - Do you need a moment alone?

¿Puedo traerle algo de beber? - PWEH-doh trah-ER-leh AHL-goh deh beh-BEHR - May I bring you something to drink?

Mis condolencias - mees kon-doh-LEN-see-ahs - My condolences

Descanse en paz - des-KAN-seh en pahs - Rest in peace

Es un honor cuidar de él/ella - es oon oh-NOR kwee-DAR deh el/EH-yah - It is an honor to care for him/her

Estoy aquí para lo que necesite - es-TOY ah-KEE PAH-rah loh keh neh-seh-SEE-teh - I am here for whatever you need

¿Le gustaría que recemos? - leh goos-tah-REE-ah keh reh-SEH-mos - Would you like us to pray?

Un abrazo fuerte - oon ah-BRAH-soh FWEHR-teh - A big hug

¿Hay alguien a quien deba llamar? - eye AHL-gyehn ah kyen DEH-bah yah-MAR - Is there someone I should call?

Cuide de usted también - KWEE-deh deh oos-TED tahm-BYEN - Take care of yourself as well

Lo siento mucho por su pérdida. - I am very sorry for your loss.

Lo siento mucho por su dolor. - I am very sorry for your pain.
Lo siento mucho por su familia. - I am very sorry for your family.
Lo siento mucho por este momento difícil. - I am very sorry for this difficult time.

Practice Dialog

Sé que estos días son muy difíciles. ¿Hay algo en lo que pueda ayudarles en este momento?

Agradecemos mucho su apoyo. ¿Podría por favor asegurarse de que tiene sus medicamentos para el dolor?

Por supuesto. Revisaré su horario de medicación de inmediato y me quedaré con ustedes un rato.

Gracias. Solo que no esté solo significa mucho para nosotros.

English translation:
I know these days are very difficult. Is there anything I can help you with right now?
We appreciate your support very much. Could you please make sure she has her pain medication?
Of course. I will check her medication schedule immediately and stay with you for a while.
Thank you. Just him not being alone means a lot to us.

Practice Scenario

La auxiliar Rosa acompañó a la familia de la señora Elena tras su fallecimiento. Les ofreció condolencia y un momento de recogimiento. Luego, con respeto, procedió con los cuidados post mórtem, bañando y vistiendo el cuerpo con suaves movimientos. Su presencia tranquila y profesional brindó consuelo a la familia en su proceso de duelo, honrando la memoria de la residente.

English translation:
The aide Rosa accompanied the family of Mrs. Elena after her passing. She offered them condolences and a moment of quiet

reflection. Then, with respect, she proceeded with post-mortem care, bathing and dressing the body with gentle movements. Her calm and professional presence provided comfort to the family in their grieving process, honoring the resident's memory.

MAINTAINING DIGNITY IN FINAL STAGES

¿Cómo se siente hoy? - KOH-moh seh SYEN-teh oy - How are you feeling today?

Voy a ayudarle - voy ah ah-yoo-DAHR-leh - I am going to help you

¿Le gustaría...? - leh goos-tah-REE-ah - Would you like...?

Vamos a... - VAH-mohs ah - Let's...

¿Está cómodo/a? - ehs-TAH KOH-moh-doh/dah - Are you comfortable?

Con permiso - kohn pehr-MEE-soh - With your permission / Excuse me

Lo/la entiendo - loh/lah en-TYEN-doh - I understand you

Gracias por su paciencia - GRAH-syahs pohr soo pah-SYEN-syah - Thank you for your patience

¿Puedo hacerle más cómodo/a? - PWEH-doh ah-SEHR-leh mahs KOH-moh-doh/dah - Can I make you more comfortable?

Su familia lo/la aprecia mucho - soo fah-MEE-lyah loh/lah ah-PREH-syah MOO-choh - Your family appreciates you very much

Estoy aquí para usted - ehs-TOY ah-KEE pah-rah oos-TEHD - I am here for you

Usted es muy importante - oos-TEHD ehs mooy eem-pohr-TAHN-teh - You are very important

Grammatical Examples

Le ofrecemos un baño caliente para su comodidad. - We offer you a warm bath for your comfort.

Le preguntamos su preferencia para el desayuno. - We ask you your preference for breakfast.

Le ayudamos a ponerse su bata favorita. - We help you put on your favorite robe.

Le escuchamos con atención cuando habla. - We listen to you attentively when you speak.

Le respetamos sus decisiones sobre su cuidado. - We respect your decisions about your care.

Practice Dialog

Voy a ayudarle a cambiarse para que esté más cómodo. ¿Le parece bien?

Sí, por favor. Quiero cooperar, pero a veces me siento muy cansado.

Lo entiendo perfectamente. Avancemos a su ritmo, sin prisa.

Gracias por su paciencia. Eso significa mucho para mí.

English translation:

I'm going to help you get changed so you're more comfortable. Is that alright with you?

Yes, please. I want to cooperate, but sometimes I feel very tired.

I understand perfectly. Let's go at your pace, no rush.

Thank you for your patience. That means a lot to me.

Practice Scenario

La Sra. García, postrada en cama, rechazaba el baño de cama. María, su auxiliar, le explicó cada paso con calma. "Ahora le voy a girar con cuidado." Usando una técnica de movilización suave y hablándole con respeto, María logró higienizarla. La Sra. García, ya cómoda y con su bata limpia, asintió con dignidad, agradecida por el cuidado compasivo que preservó su autonomía.

English translation: Mrs. García, bedridden, resisted her bed bath. María, her aide, explained each step calmly. "Now I'm going to turn you carefully." Using a gentle mobilization technique and speaking respectfully, María managed to clean her. Mrs. García, now comfortable in her clean gown, nodded with dignity, grateful for the compassionate care that preserved her autonomy.

CULTURAL AND SPIRITUAL CONSIDERATIONS

¿Cómo se siente hoy? - KOH-moh seh SYEN-teh oy - How do you feel today?

¿Necesita ayuda para rezar? - neh-seh-SEE-tah ah-YOO-dah pah-rah reh-SAHR - Do you need help to pray?

Vamos a tomar su medicina - VAH-mohs ah toh-MAHR soo meh-dee-SEE-nah - Let's take your medicine.

¿Tiene hambre o sed? - TYEH-neh AHM-breh oh sed - Are you hungry or thirsty?

¿Le gustaría escuchar música? - leh goos-tah-REE-ah es-koo-CHAHR MOO-see-kah - Would you like to listen to music?

Respeto - rehs-PEH-toh - Respect

¿Le duele aquí? - leh DWEH-leh ah-KEE - Does it hurt here?

Voy a ayudarle a bañarse - voy ah ah-yoo-DAHR-leh ah bah-NYAHR-seh - I am going to help you bathe.

¿Puedo llamar a su familia? - PWEH-doh yah-MAHR ah soo fah-MEE-lyah - May I call your family?

Comida tradicional - koh-MEE-dah trah-dee-syoh-NAHL - Traditional food

Descanso - dehs-KAHN-soh - Rest

Un momento de silencio - oon moh-MEN-toh deh see-LEN-syoh - A moment of silence

El señor García prefiere rezar en la mañana. - Mr. García prefers to pray in the morning.

La señora Vargas prefiere meditar en la tarde. - Mrs. Vargas prefers to meditate in the afternoon.

El residente prefiere una dieta vegetariana. - The resident prefers a vegetarian diet.

La residente prefiere escuchar música clásica. - The resident prefers to listen to classical music.

Los residentes prefieren celebrar las festividades. - The (male/mixed) residents prefer to celebrate the holidays.

Las residentes prefieren un ambiente tranquilo. - The (female) residents prefer a quiet environment.

Practice Dialog

¿Señora, le gustaría que recemos un rosario juntos antes de su descanso? Siempre ayuda a encontrar paz.

Sí, por favor. Rezar me da mucha fuerza, especialmente los días que duele más la artritis.

Perfecto. Voy por mis cuentas. Mientras, ¿necesita que ajuste las almohadas para estar más cómoda?

Gracias, hijo. Eres un ángel. Que Dios te bendiga por tu bondad y paciencia.

English translation:

Ma'am, would you like to pray the rosary together before your rest? It always helps to find peace.

Yes, please. Praying gives me a lot of strength, especially on days when the arthritis hurts more.

Perfect. I'll get my beads. Meanwhile, do you need me to adjust the pillows so you are more comfortable?

Thank you, my child. You are an angel. May God bless you for your kindness and patience.

Practice Scenario

La Sra. García, con demencia avanzada, se agitaba durante el baño. La auxiliar, Luisa, notó su rosario en la mesilla. "¿Le gustaría sostenerlo, señora?", preguntó suavemente. La Sra. García tomó las cuentas, sus dedos encontrando un ritmo familiar. Una calma profunda la invadió. Luisa continuó el aseo con respeto, honrando la fe que le daba paz en su confusión.

English translation: Mrs. Garcia, with advanced dementia, became agitated during her bath. The aide, Luisa, noticed her rosary on the nightstand. "Would you like to hold it, ma'am?", she asked softly. Mrs. Garcia took the beads, her fingers finding a familiar rhythm. A deep calm came over her. Luisa continued the bathing with respect, honoring the faith that gave her peace in her confusion.

RECORDING DAILY CARE NOTES

¿Cómo se siente hoy? - KOH-moh seh see-EN-teh oy - How do you feel today?

¿Necesita ayuda para ir al baño? - neh-seh-SEE-tah ah-YOO-dah pah-rah eer ahl BAH-nyoh - Do you need help going to the bathroom?

Vamos a cambiarle - BAH-mohs ah kahm-bee-AHR-leh - We are going to change you

Es hora de su medicina - ehs OH-rah deh soo meh-dee-SEE-nah - It is time for your medicine

¿Tiene dolor? - tee-EH-neh doh-LOHR - Do you have pain?

Vamos a tomar sus signos vitales - BAH-mohs ah toh-MAHR soos SEEG-nohs vee-TAH-lehs - We are going to take your vital signs

¿Tiene hambre o sed? - tee-EH-neh AHM-breh oh sed - Are you hungry or thirsty?

Voy a ayudarle a caminar - voy ah ah-yoo-DAHR-leh ah kah-mee-NAHR - I am going to help you walk

¿Le gustaría bañarse? - leh goos-tah-REE-ah bah-NYAHR-seh - Would you like to bathe?

Vamos a darle la vuelta - BAH-mohs ah DAHR-leh lah VWEHL-tah - We are going to turn you

Está todo bien - ehs-TAH TOH-doh bee-EN - Everything is okay

Descance, por favor - des-KAHN-seh pohr fah-BOHR - Rest, please

El residente está tranquilo - The resident (male) is calm.
La residente está tranquila - The resident (female) is calm.
El señor está tranquilo - The gentleman is calm.
La señora está tranquila - The lady is calm.
El paciente está tranquilo - The patient (male) is calm.
La paciente está tranquila - The patient (female) is calm.

Practice Dialog

Buenos días, ¿cómo amaneció hoy?

Muy bien, gracias. Dormí toda la noche sin molestias.

Me alegra oírlo. Voy a anotar sus signos vitales, que están dentro de lo normal.

Perfecto. ¿Me podría ayudar a tomar mi medicamento después del desayuno?

English translation:

Good morning, how did you wake up today?

Very well, thank you. I slept all night without any discomfort.

I'm glad to hear that. I'm going to note your vital signs, which are normal.

Perfect. Could you help me take my medication after breakfast?

Practice Scenario

La auxiliar anota en el gráfico: "Señora Rosa, alerta y orientada. Se quejó de dolor articular. Recibió medicamento para el dolor a las 10:00. Comió el 75% del desayuno. Transferida con andador al sillón. Pañal mojado, cambiado con piel intacta. Participó en la actividad de musicoterapia. Se le ofreció hidratación frecuente."

English translation:

The aide notes on the chart: "Mrs. Rosa, alert and oriented. Complained of joint pain. Received pain medication at 10:00. Ate 75% of breakfast. Transferred with walker to chair. Diaper wet, changed with skin intact. Participated in music therapy activity. Offered frequent hydration."

REPORTING TO NURSES AND SUPERVISORS

¿Cómo se siente hoy? - KOH-moh seh SYEN-teh oy - How are you feeling today?

Necesito reportar un cambio - neh-seh-SEE-toh reh-por-TAR oon KAM-byoh - I need to report a change

El/La señor(a) [Last Name] - el / lah seh-NYOR / seh-NYO-rah - Mr./Mrs. [Last Name]

No comió toda la comida - noh koh-MYOH TOH-dah lah koh-MEE-dah - He/She did not eat all the food

Tuvo dolor - TOO-boh doh-LOHR - He/She had pain

Se cayó - seh kah-YOH - He/She fell

Está inquieto(a) - ehs-TAH in-KYEH-toh(tah) - He/She is restless

Necesita ayuda para ir al baño - neh-seh-SEE-tah ah-YOO-dah pah-rah eer ahl BAH-nyoh - He/She needs help to go to the bathroom

Signos vitales - SEEG-nohs vee-TAH-lehs - Vital signs

Tiene fiebre - TYEH-neh FYEH-breh - He/She has a fever

No está respirando bien - noh ehs-TAH rehs-pee-RAN-doh byen - He/She is not breathing well

Refusa la medicina - reh-FOO-sah lah meh-dee-SEE-nah - He/She is refusing the medicine

El señor García necesita ayuda para levantarse. - Mr. Garcia needs help to get up.

La señora Martínez necesita ayuda para levantarse. - Mrs. Martinez needs help to get up.

El residente necesita ayuda para levantarse. - The (male) resident needs help to get up.

La residente necesita ayuda para levantarse. - The (female) resident needs help to get up.

Mi paciente necesita ayuda para levantarse. - My patient needs help to get up.

Practice Dialog

La Sra. Gutiérrez ha tenido un cambio en su estado. Noté que está más confundida hoy y no quiso comer el desayuno.

Voy a notificar al supervisor y luego revisaremos sus signos vitales. ¿Podría intentar ofrecerle el batido nutricional en media hora?

Sí, claro. Me quedo con ella. También avisaré a su hija para informarle de la situación.

Perfecto. Gracias por tu vigilancia. La comunicación temprana es clave para manejar estos cambios.

English translation:

Mrs. Gutiérrez has had a change in her condition. I noticed she is more confused today and did not want to eat her breakfast.

I will notify the supervisor and then we will check her vital signs. Could you try to offer her the nutritional shake in half an hour?

Yes, of course. I will stay with her. I will also call her daughter to inform her of the situation.

Perfect. Thank you for your vigilance. Early communication is key to managing these changes.

Practice Scenario

La auxiliar reporta a la enfermera supervisor: "La Sra. González tiene una úlcera por presión en el saco, estadío dos. Se queja de dolor. Rechazó el desayuno pero tomó sus líquidos. Está inquieta y necesita cambio de pañal. Sugiero evaluar para ajustar su plan de cuidado y el manejo del dolor". La enfermera asiente y revisa la historia clínica.

English translation:
The aide reports to the charge nurse: "Mrs. Gonzalez has a stage two pressure ulcer on her sacrum. She complains of pain. She refused breakfast but drank her fluids. She is restless and needs a diaper change. I suggest an evaluation to adjust her care plan and pain management." The nurse nods and reviews the chart.

COMMUNICATING
WITH DOCTORS

Key Vocabulary

¿Cómo se siente hoy? - KOH-moh seh see-EN-teh oy - How are you feeling today?

¿Tiene dolor? - tee-EH-neh doh-LOHR - Are you in pain?

¿Dónde le duele? - DOHN-deh leh doo-EH-leh - Where does it hurt?

Vamos a tomar la presión - VAH-mohs ah toh-MAHR lah preh-see-ON - We are going to take your blood pressure

Necesita tomar su medicina - neh-seh-SEE-tah toh-MAHR soo meh-dee-SEE-nah - You need to take your medicine

¿Puede caminar? - PWEH-deh kah-mee-NAHR - Can you walk?

Voy a ayudarle - voy ah ah-yoo-DAHR-leh - I am going to help you

¿Tiene sed? - tee-EH-neh sed - Are you thirsty?

¿Tiene hambre? - tee-EH-neh AHM-breh - Are you hungry?

¿Necesita usar el baño? - neh-seh-SEE-tah oo-SAHR el BAH-nyoh - Do you need to use the bathroom?

Respire profundamente - reh-SPEE-reh pro-foon-dah-MEN-teh - Breathe deeply

Gracias, señora/señor - GRAH-see-ahs, seh-NYOH-rah/seh-NYOHR - Thank you, ma'am/sir

Grammatical Examples

¿Le duele la cabeza? - Does your head hurt?

¿Le duele el brazo? - Does your arm hurt?

¿Le duele la espalda? - Does your back hurt?

155

¿Le duelen las piernas? - Do your legs hurt?
¿Le duelen las rodillas? - Do your knees hurt?

Practice Dialog

Buenos días, señora. ¿Cómo amaneció hoy? ¿Le duele algo?

Un poco la espalda, pero no tanto como ayer. ¿Podría ayudarme a sentarme?

Por supuesto. Vamos despacio. ¿Le parece bien si después revisamos sus signos vitales?

Sí, claro. Gracias por su ayuda, es muy amable.

English translation:

Good morning, ma'am. How are you feeling today? Does anything hurt?

My back a little, but not as much as yesterday. Could you help me sit up?

Of course. Let's go slowly. Would it be alright if we check your vital signs afterwards?

Yes, of course. Thank you for your help, you are very kind.

Practice Scenario

La señora García, con demencia avanzada, no verbalizaba su dolor. Su auxiliar de enfermería notó su expresión facial y quejidos. Le preguntó usando palabras sencillas y revisó sus signos vitales. Comunicó sus observaciones claramente a la enfermera, describiendo los cambios en su comportamiento. Esto permitió ajustar su plan de cuidado y aliviar su malestar de manera oportuna.

English translation:

Mrs. Garcia, with advanced dementia, did not verbalize her pain. Her nursing assistant noticed her facial expression and moans. She asked her using simple words and checked her vital signs. She communicated her observations clearly to the nurse, describing the changes in her behavior. This allowed them to adjust her care plan and relieve her discomfort promptly.

INSURANCE AND HEALTHCARE COORDINATION

Key Vocabulary

¿Necesita ayuda? - neh-seh-SEE-tah ah-YOO-dah - Do you need help?

Vamos a tomar su medicina - VAH-mohs ah toh-MAHR soo meh-dee-SEE-nah - Let's take your medicine

¿Dónde le duele? - DOHN-deh leh doo-EH-leh - Where does it hurt?

¿Tiene dolor? - tee-EH-neh doh-LOHR - Are you in pain?

Vamos al baño - VAH-mohs ahl BAH-nyoh - Let's go to the bathroom

Tome agua - TOH-meh AH-gwah - Drink water

¿Puede respirar profundamente? - PWEH-deh reh-spee-RAHR proh-foon-dah-MEN-teh - Can you breathe deeply?

Es hora de comer - ehs OH-rah deh koh-MEHR - It's time to eat

¿Se cayó? - seh kah-YOH - Did you fall?

Le voy a bañar - leh voy ah bah-NYAHR - I am going to bathe you

¿Tiene su tarjeta de seguro? - tee-EH-neh soo tar-HEH-tah deh seh-GOO-roh - Do you have your insurance card?

Necesito llamar a su familia - neh-seh-SEE-toh yah-MAHR ah soo fah-MEE-lee-ah - I need to call your family

Grammatical Examples

La enfermera coordina la cita. - The nurse coordinates the appointment.

El médico coordina la cita. - The doctor coordinates the appointment.
El trabajador social coordina la cita. - The social worker coordinates the appointment.
La familia coordina la cita. - The family coordinates the appointment.
El especialista coordina la cita. - The specialist coordinates the appointment.
La asistente coordina la cita. - The aide coordinates the appointment.

Practice Dialog

Ya llamé a su seguro para autorizar las visitas de terapia física.
Perfecto, ¿sabe si tienen un límite de sesiones por año?
Sí, autorizaron doce sesiones. Empezaremos la próxima semana.
Gracias por ocuparse de esto. Es un alivio no tener que hacer esas llamadas.

English translation:
I already called your insurance to authorize the physical therapy visits.
Perfect, do you know if they have a session limit per year?
Yes, they authorized twelve sessions. We will start next week.
Thank you for taking care of this. It's a relief not to have to make those calls.

Practice Scenario

La auxiliar Rosa revisa la póliza del seguro del residente. Coordina con la enfermera para autorizar una cita con el terapeuta físico. Confirman la cobertura para la terapia y el nuevo andador. Rosa documenta todo con precisión, asegurando que el señor López reciba su equipamiento médico sin demora, manteniendo su movilidad y seguridad dentro del centro de cuidados.

English translation:
The aide Rosa reviews the resident's insurance policy. She

coordinates with the nurse to authorize an appointment with the physical therapist. They confirm coverage for the therapy and the new walker. Rosa documents everything accurately, ensuring Mr. López receives his medical equipment without delay, maintaining his mobility and safety within the care center.

SHIFT CHANGE INFORMATION SHARING

Key Vocabulary

Cambio de turno - KAHM-byoh deh TOOR-noh - Shift change

Informe del turno - een-FOR-meh del TOOR-noh - Shift report

¿Cómo pasó la noche? - KOH-moh pah-SOH lah NOH-cheh - How was the night?

¿Comió y bebió bien? - koh-MYOH ee beh-BYOH byen - Did they eat and drink well?

Fue al baño - fweh ahl BAH-nyoh - They went to the bathroom

Estado de ánimo - ehs-TAH-doh deh AH-nee-moh - Mood

Señor/Señora - seh-NYOR/seh-NYOH-rah - Mr./Mrs.

¿Necesita ayuda? - neh-seh-SEE-tah ah-YOO-dah - Do you need help?

Dormir - dor-MEER - To sleep

Caída - kah-EE-dah - Fall

Toma de signos vitales - TOH-mah deh SEEG-nohs vee-TAH-lehs - Vital signs check

Medicamento - meh-dee-kah-MEN-toh - Medication

Grammatical Examples

La Sra. García tomó su medicamento. - Mrs. Garcia took her medicine.

El Sr. López tomó su medicamento. - Mr. Lopez took his medicine.

Los residentes tomaron su medicamento. - The residents took

their medicine.

La residente nueva tomó su medicamento. - The new resident (female) took her medicine.

El residente nuevo tomó su medicamento. - The new resident (male) took his medicine.

Practice Dialog

Buenos días. Tu papá descansó bien, pero no quiso desayunar. Le dejé todo anotado en la hoja de turnos.

Gracias. Revisaré las notas. ¿Necesita tomar sus medicamentos pronto?

Sí, a las diez. Ya están preparados en el pastillero con un vaso de agua.

Perfecto. Me quedo con él entonces. Que tengas un buen día.

English translation:

Good morning. Your dad rested well, but he didn't want to eat breakfast. I left everything written down on the shift sheet.

Thank you. I'll review the notes. Does he need to take his medications soon?

Yes, at ten o'clock. They're already prepared in the pill organizer with a glass of water.

Perfect. I'll stay with him then. Have a good day.

Practice Scenario

La enfermera reporta al turno nocturno: "La Sra. García tuvo una noche inquieta. Revisen su pañal cada dos horas. Se negó a tomar sus pastillas para la presión, intenten de nuevo con puré de manzana. El Sr. López necesita ayuda para transferirse al baño. Recuerden documentar todo en la hoja de registro. Buena suerte."

English translation: The nurse reports to the night shift: "Mrs. Garcia had a restless night. Check her diaper every two hours. She refused to take her blood pressure pills, try again with applesauce. Mr. Lopez needs assistance transferring to the bathroom. Remember to document everything on the flow sheet. Good luck."